T0222435

A Brief Guide to Academic Bullying

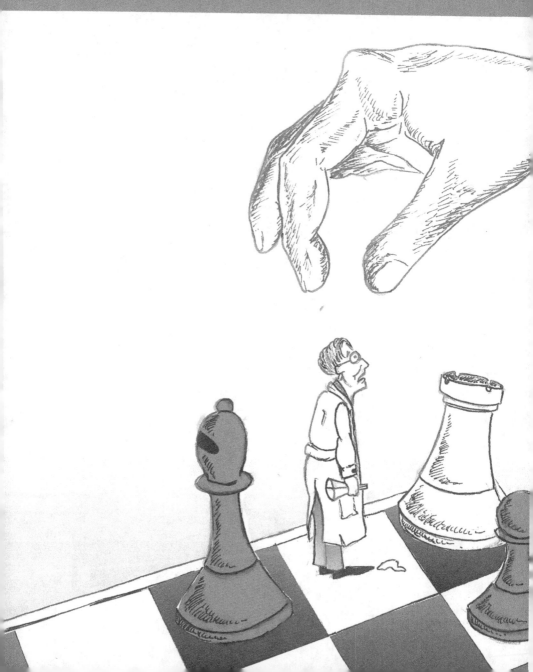

A Brief Guide to Academic Bullying

Morteza Mahmoudi

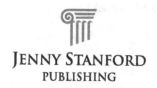

JENNY STANFORD
PUBLISHING

Published by

Jenny Stanford Publishing Pte. Ltd.
Level 34, Centennial Tower
3 Temasek Avenue
Singapore 039190

Email: editorial@jennystanford.com
Web: www.jennystanford.com

British Library Cataloguing-in-Publication Data
A catalogue record for this book is available from the British Library.

A Brief Guide to Academic Bullying

ISBN 978-981-4877-79-4 (Paperback)
ISBN 978-1-003-16034-2 (eBook)

Contents

Foreword

The educators, scientists, and researchers who crafted this book have offered their firsthand knowledge and research findings confirming that workplace bullying, academic bullying, mobbing, and even just downright abhorrent behavior compromise the lives of targets and their families (Hollis, 2017). The accounts in this book about postdoc abuse and the repercussions can leave anyone wondering if humanity has left the academic workspace. One might argue that we are witnessing a cycle of abuse. In abusive family structures, an alcoholic parent abuses a child and that child then grows up to be an alcoholic parent or a parent who enables or condones abuse. The next generation is subjected to the same unfortunate vicious cycle. The progression, unfortunately, continues until a concerted and direct intervention halts the sequence.

Analogously, we at times hear the same cycle in academic environments. In visiting various colleges and universities, I find that someone eventually admits "that's how I was treated in graduate school... I thought it was normal." Another common remark is "Oh, that's how s/he is..." as if a personality shortcoming makes the abuse tolerable. Colleagues seeking tenure and other academic advancements often hear of unnecessary battles and unwarranted competitiveness; many are told to expect the same emotional lashing in the midst of developing empirical research. In these not so hypothetical examples, leadership, faculty, and staff know where the bullies reign and stand silent in the face of maltreatment. This book reconfirms that aggression and abuse are normalized in our academic spaces.

I reflect metaphorically on a myth that many in academic leadership harbor; academics too often relate bullying and the corresponding aggressive environments to child's play in a rough house game during recess. Consequently, leaders hearing of workplace bullying often consider the behavior analogous with paper cuts or skinned knees. However, anyone who has faced years of academic bullying knows that a spritz of Bactine and band-aid does not make it all better. In the context of workplace bullying and coercion, time does not heal all wounds. What is more disconcerting, often those in power in the academy dismiss or even joke about (Hollis, 2021) stories of emotional and psychological abuse—as with all ills, simply wishing it away does not dissipate the problem.

In 1999, America witnessed a horrific landmark active shooting event at Columbine High School in Colorado. Thirteen people were killed and 20 others wounded before the two gunmen killed themselves (Mears et al., 2017). At the root of the problem, the shooters were ostracized and bullied. In the 20 years since, all 50 states have passed legislation prohibiting bullying at the K-12 level (Mezey, 2020).

From another perspective, several countries have prohibited workplace bullying. Canada, France, Finland, Sweden, Norway, France, Turkey, South Africa, and Australia, among others, recognize the dangers to both organizations and employees when bullies and tyrants undermine the workplace (Cobb, 2017). In 2021, the United States has yet to pass federal legislation protecting employees from psychological and emotional oppression regardless of race, gender, sexual orientation, religious difference, disabilities, or other protected class designations. Further, without invoking Title VII protected class designations, American employees cannot take action to combat workplace bullying unless such bullying also violates a federal statute.

Many have confirmed that bullying is an insidious behavior that damages all involved from high school sectors to international spaces. What is novel about this book is the impact on science. Research shows that bullied workers are distracted, have more health problems, and make more mistakes (Conway et al., 2021; Else, 2018). Consequently, bullied and badgered personnel working on STEM grants are at greater risk to report inaccuracies; or worse, such personnel are coerced into rushing research or falsifying data. In this context, all research team members need emotional and psychological safety to develop their best work, even if that best work yields unfavorable findings. Imagine if an engineer is rushed through structural designs, buildings and bridges could shutter, killing thousands of people. If airline pilots are rushed through training, their passengers risk their lives in flying with an under-trained or distracted pilot. Similarly, higher education executive leaders and principal investigators need to consider the public health consequences of coercion in the lab.

A Brief Guide to Academic Bullying examines a seldom discussed aspect of workplace bullying, the impact on science. With international scholars' contributions, the book opens with true academic bullying accounts in the STEM fields. The first chapter by Morteza Mahmoudi gives the reader specific examples couched within the extended duration that targets experienced the bullying and how such abuse affected their careers. Similarly, an anonymous scientist bravely shares her story and the impact on her career.

Chapters 3 and 4 by Sherry Moss analyze the social learning and normalization that evolve when the institution does not intervene to stop the bullying. Employees, professors, lab assistants, and postdocs soon recognize that bullying can be normalized, transforming the lab from a place of scientific excellence to a psychological minefield that annihilates people and the science itself. Sherry Moss also reviews how targets struggle to cope with bullying and what strategies they have used to find relief.

Chapter 5 continues with a group of writers explaining mobbing and the types of academic mobbing. Their analysis considers the departmental deterioration that occurs when workplace bullying is unchecked. This chapter also reflects on the health problems, including an example of suicide resulting from the psychological terror disseminated through workplace bullying. Chapter 6 by Krzysztof Potempa presents true accounts from targets who report workplace bullying. Consistent with the literature on this topic, Potempa reports that targets face a litany of retaliation from intrusive monitoring to job loss. The chapter also outlines how workplace bullying can evolve into a Title VII violation, sexual harassment in this case, which the United States Equal Employment Opportunity Commission (EEOC) can investigate. The authors of Chapter 7 offer various solutions inclusive of conducting further studies on academic bullying, policy development to prohibit academic bullying, academic publishers' possible role to address bullying, and institutional responsibility to create an emotionally safe lab.

We have made progress in the last 20 years with more countries prohibiting workplace bullying. Nonetheless, I recall the mercurial path women traveled to ensure that sexual harassment is prohibited in the American context. Initially, in 1964 Title VII Civil Rights laws were passed to prohibit discrimination on the basis of sex/gender. However, in the 1970s, women began filing lawsuits to prohibit sexual harassment, which was not originally accepted as a Title VII violation. The courts ruled *in Barnes v. Train (1974)* and *Tomkins v. PSE&G (1977)* that a supervisor's personal attraction to a woman on the job, and the aggression that ensued, was not covered under Title VII (Crawford, 1994). Courts disputed such arguments for over a decade through *Williams v. Saxbe (1976)* and *Brown v. City of Guthrie (1980)*.

In 1986, the Supreme Court Case *Meritor Savings Bank v. Vinson* began a change in legal perspectives when the courts ruled that women should not be burdened by a hostile workplace that results from gender-based harassment (Crawford, 1994). Over 20 years lapsed since the passing of Title VII before the courts began to accept sexual harassment charges as civil rights violations.

Arguably, workplace bullying legislation is experiencing a similar yet slower trajectory to the federal government prohibiting status-free prohibition from workplace harassment. Five states, namely, California, Minnesota, Tennessee, Utah, Maryland, and the territory of Puerto Rico, have passed some form of legislation addressing workplace bullying. However, these legislations do not empower a target to take independent action against status-free abuse (Yamada, 1999). Just as the fight against sexual harassment extended for decades, the fight against workplace bullying must also continue. This book confirms that institutional well-being, research scholars, and the critical research we produce are in peril as long as power differentials are exploited and precipitating deleterious results for all parties.

Leah P. Hollis
Rutgers University, NJ, USA
March 2021

References

Cobb E. P. (2017). *Workplace Bullying and Harassment: New Developments in International Law*. Taylor & Francis.

Conway, P. M., Høgh, A., Balducci, C., and Ebbesen, D. K. (2021). Workplace bullying and mental health, in *Pathways of Job-Related Negative Behaviour*. Springer, 101–128.

Crawford, S. (1994). A brief history of sexual-harassment law. *TRAINING-NEW YORK THEN MINNEAPOLIS-*, 31, 46–46.

Else, H. (2018). Does science have a bullying problem. *Nature*, 563(7733), 616–618.

Hollis, L. P. (2015). Take the bull by the horns: Structural approach to minimize workplace bullying for women in American higher education. *Public Policy Forum. Oxford Roundtable.*

Hollis, L. P. (2017). Workplace bullying II: A civilizational shortcoming examined in a comparative content analysis. *Comparative Civilizations Review,* 77(77), 9.

Hollis, L. P. (2021). When the first among us is the worst among us: How chairs can collaborate with the provost to address workplace bullying. *The Department Chair,* 31(4), 20–21.

Mears, D. P., Moon, M. M., and Thielo, A. J. (2017). Columbine revisited: Myths and realities about the bullying–school shootings connection. *Victims & Offenders,* 12(6), 939–955.

Mezey, S. G. (2020). Transgender policymaking: The view from the states. *Publius: The Journal of Federalism,* 50(3), 494–517.

Yamada, D. C. (1999). The phenomenon of workplace bullying and the need for status-blind hostile work environment protection. *Georgetown Law Journal,* 88, 475.

Chapter 1

You Are a Target, Not a Victim

Morteza Mahmoudi
Michigan State University, USA
mahmou22@msu.edu

Are you a target of academic incivility? Can't decide to fight or flight? Do you fear from retaliation? Well, you are not alone! This chapter is aimed to provide you (i) the minimum required information about academic bullying and its root causes and (ii) some key lessons to protect your future careers and mental health.

1.1 What Is Workplace Bullying?

Workplace bullying spans a wide spectrum of actions, including the following:

- (i) Verbal abuse—such as demeaning personal attacks
- (ii) Public shaming—can be in person in a meeting, via group email, or social media
- (iii) Isolation—being cut off from colleagues/mentors who can support you

A Brief Guide to Academic Bullying
Edited by Morteza Mahmoudi
Copyright © 2022 Jenny Stanford Publishing Pte. Ltd.
ISBN 978-981-4877-79-4 (Paperback), 978-1-003-16034-2 (eBook)
www.jennystanford.com

According to Einarsen and colleagues,[1] workplace bullying is the behavior that occurs regularly (not just once) and over a period of time (at least 6 months). The behavior may consist of harassing, offending, or isolating someone, which can directly affect their work tasks.

This is vastly different from appropriate academic discussion, feedback, and scientific criticism (none of which involve personal attacks) and is also unlike direct forthright approach and disagreement which are key components of academic freedom.

1.2   What Is Academic Bullying?

The tactics of academic bullying overlap with workplace bullying but may result in consequences unique to the academic environment such as:[1,2]

1. violations of intellectual property,
2. unfair crediting of authors, and
3. coercion to sign away authorship and/or intellectual property rights.[3-7]

Details on the types and variety of academic bullying can be found in the following short video:
https://www.youtube.com/watch?v=lKUONMm-pWo&t=4s

1.3   What Is Academic Freedom?

Academic freedom is the ability to express one's opinions and debate intellectual concepts without the fear of reprisal, including a safe space in which to conduct research in any field and draw new conclusions.

Academic freedom allows pursuit of any desired ethically sound research and includes the right to respectfully challenge or criticize any hypothesis. The right to critique someone's work is a two-way street, where dialogue generated by two individuals with academic freedom can aid in offering different perspectives and ideas as well as help with problem-solving and polishing work. Often, however, this concept is used to justify inappropriate behaviors.

There is a clear, if not intuitive, line between academic bullying (see above) and academic freedom despite unethical leaders who intentionally justify their inappropriate behaviors as academic freedom.

There is also a clear distinction between bullying and the Socratic method (when done correctly). The **Socratic method** is a form of dialogue between individuals. It is based on asking increasingly complex questions to stimulate critical thinking and to draw out ideas and underlying presuppositions. Although there are advantages and disadvantages to this method of education, it is still widely used and is not a form of bullying when done correctly and intentionally.

1.4   Most Common Examples of Academic Bullying

Examples may help to illustrate the defined behaviors (e.g., workplace bullying, academic bullying, and freedom). Please find below some examples for clarification.[2,3,8-12] Real stories from targets are presented in Chapters 2 and 4.

Abusive supervisor

- Ridicules me
- Tells me my thoughts or feelings are stupid
- Gives me the silent treatment
- Puts me down in front of others
- Invades my privacy
- Reminds me of my past mistakes and failures
- Doesn't give me credit for jobs requiring a lot of effort
- Blames me to save himself/herself from embarrassment
- Breaks promises he/she makes
- Expresses anger at me when he/she is mad for another reason
- Makes negative comments about me to others
- Is rude to me
- Does not allow me to interact with my coworkers
- Tells me I'm incompetent
- Lies to me

Academic bully

- Gives bad recommendation
- Cancels (or threatens to cancel) visa
- Interferes in job offers
- Abuses authorship
- Lengthens stay in lab
- Takes away funding
- Encourages others to mistreat target
- Uses target data without acknowledging contribution
- Cancels (or threatens to cancel) position
- Forces target to sign away rights

Bullying at the institutional level

- Cover up bullying
- Continue to elevate bullies
- Encourage code of silence
- Fail to support lab change

1.5   Root Causes of Academic Bullying

The root causes that plant the seeds for academic bullying incidents and more information on the reasons behind abusive behaviors are provided in Chapter 3:

(i) The current research ecosystems are in favor of bullies to thrive; according to Dr. Moss, "Working conditions in academic labs encourage abusive supervision. It is time to improve monitoring of and penalties for abuse."[3]

(ii) There is a confusion over the concepts of academic freedom and academic bullying. Although unethical leaders intentionally justify their inappropriate behaviors as academic freedom, there is a clear and intuitive line between academic bullying and academic freedom (see Section 1.3 for details). Academic bullying is when leaders use verbal abuse, such as ridiculing students, public shaming, isolation, silent treatment, and academic threatening such as visa cancellation or giving a bad recommendation. At the institutional level, it means covering up for the bullies or forcing targets to use code of silence. More details on differences between academic bullying and academic freedom are available through our recent podcast at Michigan State University: https://podcasts.apple.com/us/podcast/morteza-mahmoudi-and-barbara-roberts-on-academic-bullying/id1480014096?i=1000467238613

(iii) Academic bullies are clever! They know how to pressure students over the phone or in private meeting to minimize the trace of their actions.[13] When targets do not have any documentation as evidence to back up the bullying behavior against them to present to an investigation committee, it means the bullying incidents never happened. Incidents that are not in writing are not substantial evidence to warrant investigation in most institutions. In severe cases, unethical leaders may force targets to sign away their rights to intellectual property and authorship.[13] International scholars are more vulnerable to these actions due to their unstable visa status compiled with their cultural and language barriers.

(iv) Currently, there are no official regulations in the academic world to help prevent academic bullying and protect targets. The simple word about the current legislation is that "academic bullying is unethical and inappropriate, but **it is not illegal** unless it can be tide up to discrimination and sexual harassment." The issues presented by academic bullying urgently need consideration by legislators. There is a significant effort in the United States to pass bills on health in the workplace (e.g., efforts by Yamada[14]). However, in addition to the complexities involved in addressing workplace bullying, academic bullying in higher education requires broader regulations. For example, a large portion of postdocs are international (more than 50% in 2015, according to a report by the US National Science Foundation[15]) and, at least during the course of their current investigation, must protect their visa from cancellation, which is frequently the leverage bullies use to enforce silence. If appropriate new laws are crafted, universities may implement the same zero-tolerance policy that exists for sexual harassment, especially if they believe their reputation to be in danger and can be legally sued by targets of bullying. Institutions may then be motivated to provide training programs for both faculty members and students. In the presence of zero-tolerance policies, institutional leaders would be more alert to the consequences of unethical behavior and thus less likely to tolerate them. It bears repeating that these strategies will not be effective unless all stakeholders work together in an integrated fashion; in the related area of sexual harassment, the National Academies of Sciences, Engineering, and Medicine has weighed in on the insufficient effects of regulations and policies alone on a significant reduction in the number of incidents.[16]

(v) The psychological knowledge in helping the targets of academic bullying is not available. There is little known about the effects of academic bullying on targets, their work, and their personal lives. The simplest analogy for this issue is the emergence of diseases related to e-cigarettes; a few months ago, the first death related to e-cigarettes was reported and confirmed in the United States. The issue is that, unlike cigar, the types of lung diseases caused by e-cigarettes are not known and there are no established cures for them. Similarly, the psychological knowledge about the effects of academic bullying and how to help targets has not been uncovered yet!

(vi) There are serious problems in fair and unbiased internal investigations of academic bullying incidents by institutions.[9] In the absence of a global committee to audit the reports of academic bullying, institutions may not conduct unbiased investigations due to several reasons, including their reputation, limited options to offer the targets, the bully's influence on the investigation, and the powerless nature of targets.

(vii) The outcomes of the internal investigations by academic institutions are confidential. When the outcomes are not publicly available,[17] there is no accountability pressure on the members of the investigation committee to be completely unbiased and fair.

(viii) Targets develop willingness to tolerate abusive behaviors due to many reasons; one of them is the limited number of positions in high-ranked universities. A simple analogy to better understand the reason behind the willingness to tolerate unacceptable behaviors: according to the concept of market equilibrium, the only fair condition for both buyers and sellers is when there is neither excess demand nor excess supply. Otherwise, one of the parties is forced to enter the exchange, receiving less of the service or profit they desire. This condition exists in the case of students and scholars who are eager to work in high-ranked institutions where there are a limited number of positions. This means that lab members can be easily replaced by other candidates. This pressure, and the expendable sentiment, causes a willingness to tolerate bullying among targets. It is easy to imagine, as a target, that you are easily replaceable if you "rock the boat" or cause "trouble" for drawing attention to serious issues in the workplace. There are many other critical reasons, including fear of retaliation, mobbing, and visa cancellation.

The unfortunate reality is that mild incidents of academic bullying such as insults, snubs, and invasions of privacy by lab leaders are now considered as a norm in many high-ranking universities. Even at the higher level and with more serious types of bullying, which can include violations of intellectual property and unfair crediting of authors in scientific publications, targets are hesitant to speak up due to several reasons including less trust to the fair and unbiased investigation by the institutions.

1.6   How to Protect Yourself Against Bullying Behaviors?

(i) Try to read the following important books; which can provide you with essential skills and knowledge to manage the situation appropriately and develop a strong plan to oppose academic bullies and their networks:
    - *Influence: The Psychology of Persuasion* by Robert B. Cialdini
    - *7 Habits of Highly Effective People* by Stephen R. Covey
    - *Designing Your Life: How to Build a Well-Lived, Joyful Life* by Bill Burnett and Dave Evans

- *Unfu*k Yourself: Get Out of Your Head and into Your Life* by Gary John Bishop

(ii) "Try to document and record your interactions, including the abusive behavior. This can be accomplished by saving emails, writing memos to document verbal conversations, or making sure to have conversations in the presence of a trusted ally. Having organized documentation relating to specific incidences not only can help strengthen your case, but can also help you keep incidences fresh in your mind.

(iii) Consult your institution's ombudsman or mediation office. The professionals there, trained in dealing with harassment and bullying, will listen to your issue and offer guidance. Often, they are not able to act on your behalf or prevent the behaviors from happening, but they can advise you on the best course of action. Many times, simply having a listening ear with helpful resources can be a critical point in many cases.

(iv) One important piece of advice is to insist that the institution provide a summary letter of their findings on your complaint case. With that in place, if any future employer has a question about what happened, you have evidence that your claims were upheld by an investigation and there was no wrongdoing on your part. However, be aware that such a summary may also include negative or unsubstantiated testimony regarding your own actions, which could damage your reputation.

(v) Look for others who might be experiencing the same situation but are afraid of speaking up. Band together, document your stories, and amass evidence. It is much more difficult for an institution to ignore or brush away the concerns of multiple researchers who present their case together. There is strength and validity in numbers, which may allow targets to share their stories who otherwise may not be able to do so.

(vi) Have an exit strategy in mind, ideally in advance. This may be another position in a different laboratory group, department, or even institution. Importantly, this may mean cultivating other mentors and collaborators well in advance so that you can ask them for recommendation letters.

(vii) Starting the moment you decide to speak up, you should be prepared for retaliation. Think through all the potential consequences of speaking up, which may range from tainting your reputation to being fired or even an increase in bullying behavior. Even a well-founded complaint documenting a clear history of abuse may elicit strong institutional resistance. Having another job to move to—with the financial security it brings—will give you leverage to lodge a full complaint against the bully. Importantly, this may mean cultivating other mentors and collaborators well in advance so that you can ask them for recommendation letters.

(viii) Sadly, targets of bullying often underestimate how well connected a bully is or how much political or financial sway he may hold over a department or an institution. Therefore, you also need to consider some additional actions by bullies described in Chapters 5 and 6 in more detail.

(ix) Just as with cycles of domestic abuse, so too can the bullied become the next bully in academia. Therefore, try to heal your wounds to avoid that fate! Instead, to heal the wounds inflicted upon you, you can write about the problem of academic bullying and share your experiences with others to help them out.

(x) And my last piece of advice: remind yourself that you are a target, not a victim. Just like targets of sexual harassment, you did nothing wrong to bring on this bad behavior, and it is not your fault. It is important to remember that you got to your position by hard work and scientific talent. Have confidence to stand up to your bully—by finding allies, drawing on institutional resources, and reclaiming your rights."[18]

Ultimately, of course, the only effective way to stop the chain of academic bullying is for the entire scientific workforce to decide that bullying will no longer be tolerated in our workplaces. All possible approaches to conduct such an effective way are summarized in Chapter 7.

1.7 Conclusions

Targets of bullying are often the most vulnerable members of the scientific workforce—they may be low-paid graduate students or postdocs, living in a foreign country, navigating a foreign language and culture, and whose immigration status is tied directly to their employment. They may also have young families, be living paycheck to paycheck, and have health insurance and other benefits that depend on a contract position that can be revoked with little to no notice or cause. Finally, targets on the low end of a power differential are not likely to be supported by their institutions, particularly institutions that rely on the big grant earnings brought in by senior "bullies." A brief definition on abusive behaviors, their root causes, and possible strategies that can be used by the targets to help themselves are provided in this chapter.

References

1. Einarsen, S., Hoel, H., Cooper, C., *Bullying and Emotional Abuse in the Workplace: International Perspectives in Research and Practice*. CRC Press: 2003.

2. Tepper, B. J., Consequences of abusive supervision. *Academy of Management Journal*, 2000, 43(2), 178–190.

3. Moss, S., Research is set up for bullies to thrive. *Nature*, 2018, 560, 529–529.

4. Mahmoudi, M., Poorman, J. A., Silver, J. K., Representation of women among scientific Nobel Prize nominees. *The Lancet*, 2019, 394(10212), 1905–1906.

5. Tepper, B. J., Moss, S. E., Lockhart, D. E., Carr, J. C., Abusive supervision, upward maintenance communication, and subordinates' psychological distress. *Academy of Management Journal*, 2007, 50(5), 1169–1180.

6. Twale, D. J., *Understanding and Preventing Faculty-on-Faculty Bullying: A Psycho-Social-Organizational Approach*. Routledge: 2017.

7. Jones, B., Hwang, E., Bustamante, R. M., African American female professors' strategies for successful attainment of tenure and promotion at predominately White institutions: It can happen. *Education, Citizenship and Social Justice*, 2015, 10(2), 133–151.

8. Smith, D. K., The race to the bottom and the route to the top. *Nature Chemistry*, 2020, 12(2), 101–103.

9. Mahmoudi, M., Improve reporting systems for academic bullying. *Nature*, 2018, 562(7728), 494–494.

10. Mahmoudi, M., Ameli, S., Moss, S., The urgent need for modification of scientific ranking indexes to facilitate scientific progress and diminish

academic bullying. *BioImpacts*, 2019, 10(1), 5–7. doi: 10.15171/bi.2019.30.

11. Mahmoudi, M., Moss, S., Scarcity of lab positions in high-ranked institutions creates a breeding ground for bullies. *BioImpacts*, 2019, 9(4), 251.

12. Mahmoudi, M., Moss, S. E., Tie institutions' reputations to their anti-bullying record. *Nature*, 2019, 572(7770), 439–439.

13. Mahmoudi, M., Academic bullies leave no trace. *BioImpacts*, 2019, 9, 129–130.

14. Wang, P., Yoo, B., Yang, J., Zhang, X., Ross, A., Pantazopoulos, P., Dai, G., Moore, A., GLP-1R–targeting magnetic nanoparticles for pancreatic islet imaging. *Diabetes*, 2014, 63(5), 1465–1474.

15. Monopoli, M. P., Åberg, C., Salvati, A., Dawson, K. A., Biomolecular coronas provide the biological identity of nanosized materials. *Nature Nanotechnology*, 2012, 7(12), 779.

16. The National Academies of Sciences, Engineering, and Medicine (Consensus Study Report), *Sexual Harassment of Women: Climate, Culture, and Consequences in Academic Sciences, Engineering, and Medicine*. The National Academies Press, Washington DC: 2018.

17. Abbott, A., Germany's prestigious Max Planck Society conducts huge bullying survey. *Nature*, 2019, 571(7763), 14–15.

18. Mahmoudi, M., A survivor's guide to academic bullying. *Nature Human Behaviour*, 2020, 4(11), 1091.

Chapter 2

A Sample Target Story

Maria Smith*

My story begins as an assistant professor in my home country, during which time I also held visiting professorships at prominent research universities in Europe and the United States. I had successfully developed a technology with the potential to diagnose human diseases and I had both published and patented my work.

In 2015, I reached out to a renowned group of researchers at a prestigious research institution to see if I could collaborate with them to translate my technology for clinical use. They invited me to give a job talk for a position within their group.

Afterward, one senior principal investigator (PI) in the group offered me a postdoctoral position within his group, with the promise of a quick promotion to a more independent position to follow. This should have been my first red flag warning.

However, I was quickly promoted to instructor within his group. I oversaw three postdoctoral researchers and took over much of the grant writing for the lab. In addition, my supervisor asked me to do

---

*The author does not wish to disclose additional information (including affiliation and email).

A Brief Guide to Academic Bullying
Edited by Morteza Mahmoudi
Copyright © 2022 Jenny Stanford Publishing Pte. Ltd.
ISBN 978-981-4877-79-4 (Paperback), 978-1-003-16034-2 (eBook)
www.jennystanford.com

some very unprofessional, personal things for him such as editing photos of his family, writing his promotion letters, creating an overly flattering Wikipedia page for him, and nominating him for awards. These should have been the second big red flag.

At the same time, this PI was very encouraging about translating my technology into a diagnostic test for clinical applications and together we submitted a patent for this idea. About one year after I joined the lab, he and I had an explosive disagreement about who should get senior authorship of a publication related to my diagnostic test, all of the experimental work and analysis for which had been done prior to joining his group.

At this point, the full-on harassment began. He called me at home on my cell phone and even sometimes late at night. He wanted details about the technology, but scolded me for putting them into emails. (I didn't know it at the time, but he was secretly starting a company based on my technology.)

Throughout the next year, a pattern of bullying behaviors emerged in our in-person or phone meetings. He used all the bully's tactics: berating, shouting profanity, attempting to humiliate me in front of colleagues, and threatening to terminate my job among other things. Nearly all of these happened behind closed doors.

But I put up with these behaviors because I was succeeding in my science. Our patent was filed and I had won an internal university grant for $300,000. He had promised to help me get promoted to an assistant professor position.

Instead, during a time when my supervisor was away on sabbatical, I received a one-two sucker punch to the gut: a letter terminating my position due to a "lack" of funding and a request for access to my raw data from the company that my supervisor had set up based on my patented technology without my knowledge.

In an email, I confronted the PI and asked for an explanation. At the same time, I contacted my institution's ombudsman office and a top administrator to find out what my options were. My stress and anxiety levels were through the roof. In an instant it seemed that I might no longer have a job or health insurance at a time when we were starting our family.

As I refused to respond to his continued phone calls, my PI flew back from his sabbatical and requested a meeting in his office. I did not feel physically safe meeting in his office, and so we met in a public coffee shop off campus. Another red flag. When I confronted him, he threw an emotional fit, which flowed from rage to tears. He brought up the assistant professor promotion again and even dangled the idea of bringing me into the company.

At the time, I decided to take a forgiving approach. But in hindsight, he was simply manipulating me. Later, I would learn he had a pattern of behaving badly and then begging for forgiveness and promising to do better. Too often, academic bullying is akin to having an abusive domestic partner—one who has more financial and political power over you and uses it against you.

Two years after joining the bully's research group, I was promoted to a fully independent position, with my own designated laboratory and office space, and I would report to the department chair. I also won two more prestigious internal grants. My new independence and success had me feeling secure, but my former supervisor had also been promoted to the head of the institutional center that housed our labs, still casting a menacing shadow over my work.

Over the next six months, I developed a new technology that improved upon the first diagnostic test and filed a patent for it. When my former PI somehow found out, he started asking for a meeting and questions about it. When I met him in a public space on campus, he again threw an ugly scene, yelling at me that he should share in the patent.

Immediately, a new wave of retaliation began: text messages from colleagues pressuring me and weird, newly placed restrictions on running my lab that other assistant professors didn't share.

It was a classic bait and switch pattern of an abuser. When his bullying tactics didn't work to get what he wanted, he'd dangle an offer of career advancement. Once he had his way, he'd go right back to bullying. If I complained to a higher administrator, he threatened my job and promised to destroy my reputation and career chances. I was yo-yoing between humiliation, **manipulation, AND** making progress in my research and career. It was a completely unsustainable state of affairs.

By this point, I had formulated a backup plan and had applied to other assistant professor positions. When things had escalated to the point that I raised an official institutional complaint, I had a written offer from another employer.

The institution found my complaint to be valid and a pattern of bullying behavior by my former PI, yet they only chose to reprimand the bully and send him to a training course. (A tactic they had already used in the past with this professor—which had clearly failed.) My only option was to continue working in the same research center and department where this menace held a very senior position. Instead, I resigned and moved to my new institution.

Although this may seem like a bad outcome, I'm very much at peace today to be doing my science in a supportive, nonhostile environment.

Chapter 3

Causes of Abusive Supervision: The Case of Bullying in Academic Science

Sherry Moss

Wake Forest University, USA

mosss@wfu.edu

This chapter is focused on the root causes of academic bullying in higher education.

3.1 Introduction

Abusive supervision has been a significant topic of research in the field of organizational behavior since 2000. Defined as "the sustained display of hostile verbal and nonverbal behaviors, excluding physical contact,"[1] typical behaviors directed toward subordinates by supervisors include ridicule, blame, rudeness, lying, put downs, public shaming, withholding credit, invasion of privacy, and giving the silent treatment. These behaviors have been well documented in many types of organizations and between 10% and 14% of supervisors in the United States are estimated to display

A Brief Guide to Academic Bullying

Edited by Morteza Mahmoudi

Copyright © 2022 Jenny Stanford Publishing Pte. Ltd.

ISBN 978-981-4877-79-4 (Paperback), 978-1-003-16034-2 (eBook)

www.jennystanford.com

these behaviors on a regular basis.[2] The field of academic science is unique in that the estimates for abusive supervision are significantly higher. For example, a survey at the Max Planck Institute in Germany reported that 17.5% of respondents had experienced bullying at some point in their careers,[3] while 21% of PhD students in a *Nature* survey said they'd been bullied during their programs.[4] Another study[5] estimated that between 25% and 33% of individuals in academic science had been bullied in the past year, while 40% said they had witnessed a colleague being bullied.

Much is known about the consequences of abusive supervision. Consequences include negative job attitudes, such as lowered job satisfaction and organizational commitment; decreased mental health including burnout, exhaustion, tension, anxiety, and depression; and dysfunctional organizational behaviors such as deviance, retaliation, lowered performance, turnover, and work-to-family conflict.[6] The fiscal effects of these consequences have been estimated to cost U.S. organizations nearly $24 billion annually.[7]

Given the devastating and costly effects of abusive supervision, it is important to understand the antecedents, so that possible solutions or interventions can be designed. Several recent reviews of the literature and meta-analyses reveal that the antecedents fall into three main categories: (1) social learning, (2) identity threat, and (3) self-regulation impairment.[6,8,9] I will discuss each of these categories and then describe how academic science has unique characteristics that illuminate each category. I will end by examining how each of these categories relates to the power dynamics at play in academic science.

3.2 Social Learning

Social learning theory (SLT) examines the effects of role models on those around them.[10] In contrast to the operant theory, which suggests that individuals learn by acting on their environment and experiencing positive or negative consequences,[11] SLT suggests that individuals learn new behaviors by observing and imitating others.[12] They also learn from the consequences they witness being experienced by role models. For example, the observation of a father getting his way by shaming and putting down the mother may reinforce the notion in a child that this type of bullying results in positive consequences. Owing to the absence of other role models demonstrating different methods of getting their way, the child may imitate the abusive parent.

In life, we have many different role models. They reside at the familial, departmental, organizational, and even cultural levels. For instance, several studies have shown that, like domestic violence, those who witness or experience violence in their families of origin are more likely to be perpetrators of abusive supervision in the workplace.[13,14] Similarly, there is ample evidence that bully bosses are important role models for direct reports, who go on to bully their own subordinates,[15] especially when they believe that abusive behavior from their own leaders is intended to strengthen performance.[16] This type of behavior is more prevalent in workplace climates where abusive supervision and hostile organizational climates are the norm.[9,15] Finally, power distance—the extent to which lower ranking individuals in a society accept and expect that power is distributed unequally[17]—provides a strong normative backdrop for abusive supervision in countries, or among individuals, with high power distance.[18]

Several of these elements of social learning are illustrated in a recent case of academic bullying at the University of Wisconsin-Madison, which ended in the suicide of a graduate student named John Brady. Brady, a doctoral candidate in the Wireless Communication and Sensing Laboratory at UW-Madison, under the direction of engineering professor Akbar Sayeed, experienced a toxic and abusive lab environment, characterized by daily rants, name-calling, tirades, exploitation, and threats. This environment was allowed to continue, presumably undetected by university leadership. They did not notice that the turnover in this lab was abnormally high, nor did they realize the devastating effects on the student well-being, having failed to investigate several complaints.[19] In an interview following the suicide of this promising young engineer, Professor Sayeed, who had secured millions of dollars in research money for the institution, admitted that his behavior was "unprofessional," suggesting that he grew up in a "militaristic environment" in Pakistan and was treated harshly by his father, which led to anger issues that he apparently projected onto his lab employees. This story illustrates how cultural differences, particularly high power distance, and familial role models strongly influence the behavior of academic bullies.

At the same time, there appears to be a prevailing attitude that "science is tough," which creates an environment that supports and reinforces bullying behavior in academic science.[20] Young scientists evaluate the social climate in which they receive their education, assessing the norms for "appropriate" behavior.[15] With this socially constructed mindset, young scientists later turn into PIs (principal investigators) who have developed the belief that if they are not tough on their students, like their own PIs who were tough with them, they will not develop the skills and work ethic necessary to survive and succeed in the field of science. This type of example illustrates both the "trickle-down" nature of academic bullying and the hostile workplace culture which often develops in labs and institutions driven by competition and the strong need for achievement in science.[20] It also suggests that, in many cases, abusive behavior is intentional and strategic, a finding which is supported in the literature from organizational behavior.[21]

3.3 Identity Threats

Individuals in positions of authority are particularly vulnerable to identity threats because holding such positions is an indication of the occupant's competence. When something or someone threatens an authority figure's sense of identity as a competent leader, they are more likely to use some form of aggression as a calculated strategy to lessen the threat.[22] For supervisors, threats may come from above, from below, or from within.[6]

3.3.1 Threats from Within

Beginning with threats from within, certain personality characteristics are accompanied by greater than average threat sensitivity. Researchers have found relationships between the "Dark Triad" personality traits (Machiavellianism, psychopathy, and narcissism) and a leader's propensity to be abusive.[23,24] In addition, supervisors with high psychological entitlement, strong individual identity, and high social dominance are more likely than others to engage in abusive supervision.[25-27] Individuals with these psychological profiles are self-oriented, making them more vulnerable to retaliate when they are confronted by others who threaten their perception of superiority over others.[6] While there is no reason to believe that scientists are any more likely to embody these dark personality characteristics than leaders in other fields, these characteristics, paired with threats from above, can lead to toxic and abusive laboratory environments.

3.3.2 Threats from Above

Threats from above come from higher level managers who apply significant pressure[34] or commit some form of injustice,[28,29] which triggers the supervisor's sense of dignity and respect. This type of threat emanating from above produces a displaced aggression, which results in the targeting of a supervisor's direct reports.[30] In the field of academic science, there is reason to believe that PIs are under significant pressure from their institutions to publish and secure grants, as they bring money and prestige to the organization.[31,33] Jennifer Lavers, a marine scientist, recounts her experience as a young researcher in being told that her grants were too small or that her published work appeared in journals with impact factors that were too low or that she was not collaborating with the right people.[34] In some cases, the pressure Lavers describes is then displaced and passed on to the PI's students and postdocs in the form of abusive supervision.[20] This phenomenon in academic science is evident in the recent news about an empathy researcher at the Max Planck Institute in Germany who created an "atmosphere of fear" in her lab, specifically targeting and mistreating pregnant female lab employees. Her own explanation for her behavior was that she "worked on the expense of my own balance," implying that she was under tremendous pressure.[35]

3.3.3 Threats from Below

Much of the research on abusive supervision has focused on the behaviors and characteristics of those who are bullied. One of the first studies to examine the antecedents of abusive supervision[36] was grounded in the literature on moral exclusion,[37] which suggests that some people are considered deserving of fair treatment while others are not. For those who fall outside of an individual's *scope of justice*, the normal rules of fair treatment do not apply and they are often mistreated. The literature on target precipitation supports this notion as well, suggesting that some followers are more provocative targets than others.[38,39] Those who appear to be weak, vulnerable, annoying or unlikable, or otherwise "high-maintenance" are more likely targets of abuse.[9,40]

According to the moral exclusion theory, there are three primary factors that are thought to be precursors to moral exclusion: dissimilarity, conflict, and utility. Using participants from seven healthcare organizations, Tepper, Moss, and Duffy (2011) demonstrated how each of these factors predicted abusive supervision.[36] It is well documented in the conflict literature that dissimilarity leads to conflict.[41] While "surface-level dissimilarity" such as gender, race, or cultural background may lead to conflict, "deep dissimilarity," or the differences in values and attitudes, has an even stronger effect on conflict.[42-44] Given the preponderance of white males in academic science[45] and the increasing percentage of women in graduate science programs[46] and foreigners in postdoc positions,[47,48] there is ample reason to suspect that both surface-level and deep dissimilarity are important factors driving abusive supervision in academic science. When dissimilarity leads to increased conflict, the probability of abuse is even higher.

Tepper and colleagues further explicate how dissimilar employees are more likely to be evaluated poorly[49] and how these poor evaluations lead supervisors to think of them as having little *utility*. When individuals are perceived as having low utility, they become provocative targets,[39] making them easy targets for aggression from the supervisor. While poor performance has been shown to be an antecedent to bullying,[36,50] it is not only the poor performers who are targeted.

Another specific study that highlights the significant role of identity threat, in terms of threats from within (i.e., personality) and threats from below, was conducted by Khan et al. (2018).[26] While replicating the finding that abusers will target low performers because they are provocative targets as suggested above, they also found that outstanding performers may be the targets of abusive supervision under specific circumstances.

In particular, they explicated the role of the supervisor's social dominance orientation—a personality trait that represents an individual's preference for hierarchy within any social system and the domination of lower status groups.[51] Khan et al. (2018) found that supervisors with high social dominance orientation were more likely to feel threatened by high performers, who may have garnered some of the resources and attention normally reserved for supervisors (e.g., praise from higher ups), and, in turn, bullied them in an effort to put them back in their proper place in the hierarchy.[26] Because white men dominate in the field of science, and also have higher than average social dominance orientation,[51] it is probable that PIs with high social dominance orientation may feel threatened by brilliant young PhD students or postdocs, particularly those who are different such as women and foreigners, and bully them so that they, themselves, are not outshined or replaced by dissimilar others. There is sufficient evidence to suspect that women[52] and foreign postdocs[47] are the most likely targets of academic bullying. This research, again, provides support for the notion that sometimes abusive supervision is cold, calculated, and strategic.[7] On the other hand, some research focuses on "hot" abuse—the kind that emanates from a lapse in self-regulation.[53]

3.4 Self-Regulation Impairment

Above I alluded to the kind of abuse that is strategic and calculated— the kind that is intended to get subordinates in line because they are performing poorly and "need" an intervention[21] or because they are performing extraordinarily well and "need" to be put back in their place.[26] However, much of the research has focused on contextual circumstances which are frustrating and aggravating and which cause supervisors to lash out, engaging in hostile behavior toward subordinates. Building on conservation of resources theory,[54] supervisors may find that certain organizational or job-related circumstances result in cognitive resource depletion, a condition that precipitates the loss of self-regulatory ability. Because supervisory jobs are difficult, requiring complex decision-making, problem-solving, and interactions with difficult people, they consume significant cognitive resources. When these conditions drain one's cognitive resources, the probability of a "hot," fatigued, unregulated response to a subordinate's provocation is high. The same German researcher mentioned above, Tania Singer, apologized "for the mistakes I made as a young director of a big Max Planck Department," claiming that "my psychological and physical resources are exhausted."[35]

While these hot episodes may be more likely to occur due to acute workload pressure, injustice from above, or other circumstances, they are particularly likely when the supervisor has not had proper sleep, exercise, or is concerned with family issues.[6] Finally, the tendency to lash out at subordinates is even more likely when these circumstances are accompanied by trait-like self-regulatory ability deficits, such as low emotional intelligence, trait self-control, political skill, or mindfulness. [6,24]

3.5 Power Dynamics

When putting all of these causes together, it becomes obvious that academic science embodies a number of characteristics that enhance the probability of bullying. These characteristics result in huge power differentials between researchers and students, creating toxic environments in which bullying is likely to thrive.[33] First, the eager graduate students and postdocs clamber to join the most prestigious programs with the most prolific researchers,[55] hoping to have their best shot at solving the important problems of the world and making their marks on science. Famous, admired scientists are strong magnets for the most talented of these young scientists, who assign them rock star status. Further, the importance of their work (e.g., cancer research) gives some scientists an even loftier, high-profile status, garnering even more power and figurative distance from their underlings.[31] The importance of their work can be so heady that it overshadows their concerns about basic humanity and appropriate treatment of subordinates. Students may even put up with mistreatment as an unwelcome, but inevitable side effect of working in a famous researcher's lab.[4]

In addition, researchers have significant reward and coercive power over their lab members.[56] Students' reliance on powerful PIs to give (or take away) resources such as funding, letters of recommendation, and opportunities to publish creates an unhealthy dependence, making it that much harder to leave a supervisor's lab and start over somewhere else.[52] Students who complain end up with tarnished reputations and few prospects for continuing their education, making the "code of silence" a more attractive and likely response to bullying.[4,55]

Getting further into the identity threat territory, there is an important confluence of human capital in the scientific fields. First, the field has historically been dominated by white males.[57] Currently, however, the face of the field is changing as the ranks of PhD programs and postdoc appointments are filled with dissimilar others—specifically women[58] and foreigners.[59] As per the discussion above, dissimilarity is an important precursor to moral exclusion, meaning dissimilar others are more likely to be provocative targets of abuse.[36] Combine this tendency with high social dominance orientation where majority and higher status individuals feel threatened by the success of dissimilar others who are hierarchically inferior and who appear to be becoming the majority and you have a recipe for abuse.[26]

Finally, and most concerning of all, there is the social learning element of student development. Getting their training in a lab with a famous, prolific, powerful scientist doing important work who is also an abuser sends a powerful, albeit subconscious, message that bullying is associated with success. This powerful formula makes it more likely that abusive supervision will continue in academic science unless significant interventions are implemented now, so that the future of science, and scientists, is safe.

References

1. Tepper, B. J. (2000). Consequences of abusive supervision, *Academy of Management Journal*, 43(2), pp. 178–190.

2. Schat, A. C., Frone, M. R., and Kelloway, E. K. (2006). Prevalence of workplace aggression in the U.S. workforce: Findings from a national study. In E. K. Kelloway, J. Barling, and J. J. Hurrell (Eds.), *Handbook of Workplace Violence*, pp. 47–89 (Sage Publishing, USA).

3. Abbott, A. (2019). Germany's prestigious Max Planck Society conducts huge bullying survey, *Nature*, 5, pp. 14–15.

4. Flaherty, C. (2019). Mental health, bullying, career uncertainty, *Inside Higher Ed*, November 14.

5. Keashly, L. (2018). Nature and prevalence of workplace bullying and mobbing in the US: What do the numbers mean? In M. Duffy and D. Yamada (Eds.), *Workplace Bullying and Mobbing in the U.S.* (Praeger, USA).

6. Tepper, B. J., Simon, L., and Park, H. M. (2017). Abusive supervision, *Annual Review of Organizational Psychology and Organizational Behavior*, 4, pp. 123–152.

7. Tepper, B. J., Duffy, M. K., Henle, C. A., and Lambert, L. S. (2006). Procedural injustice, victim precipitation, and abusive supervision, *Personnel Psychology*, 59(1), pp. 101–123.

8. Martinko, M. J., Harvey, P., Brees, J. R., and Mackey, J. (2013). A review of abusive supervision research, *Journal of Organizational Behavior*, 34, pp. S120–S137.

9. Zhang, Y., and Bednall, T. C. (2016). Antecedents of abusive supervision: A meta-analytic review, *Journal of Business Ethics*, 139(3), pp. 455–471.

10. Bandura, A. (1986). The explanatory and predictive scope of self-efficacy theory, *Journal of Social and Clinical Psychology*, 4, pp. 359–373.

11. Skinner, B. F. (1938). *The Behavior of Organisms: An Experimental Analysis* (Appleton-Century, USA).

12. Bandura, A. (1973). *Aggression: A Social Learning Analysis* (Prentice Hall, USA).

13. Garcia, P. R. J. M., Restubog, S. L. D., Kiewitz, C., Scott, K. L., and Tang, R. L. (2014). Roots run deep: Investigation psychological mechanisms between history of family aggression and abusive supervision, *Journal of Applied Psychology*, 99, pp. 883–897.

14. Kiewitz, C., Restobug, S. L. D., Zagenczyk, T. J., Scott, K. D., Garcia, P. R. J. M., and Tang, R. L. (2012). Sins of the parents: Self-control as a buffer between supervisors' previous experience of family undermining and subordinates' perceptions of abusive supervision, *Leadership Quarterly*, 23, pp. 869–882.

15. Mawritz, M. B., Mayer, D. M., Hoobler, J. M., Wayne, S. J., and Marinova, S. V. (2012). A trickle-down model of abusive supervision, *Personnel Psychology*, 65, pp. 325–357.

16. Liu, D., Liao, H., and Loi, R. (2012). The dark side of leadership: A three-level investigation of the cascading effect of abusive supervision on employee creativity, *Academy of Management Journal*, 55, pp. 1187–1212.

17. Hofstede, G. (1997). *The IBM Handbook of Organizational Behavior.* (Thomson Business Press, UK).

18. Vogel, R. M., Mitchell, M. S., Tepper, B. J., Restobug, S. L. D., Hu, C., et al. (2015). A cross-cultural examination of subordinates' perceptions of and reactions to abusive supervision, *Journal of Organizational Behavior,* 36, pp. 720–745.

19. Meyerhofer, K. (2019). Toxic lab lasted for years. UW-Madison had little idea until a student died by suicide, *Wisconsin State Journal,* October 31.

20. Farley, S., and Sprigg, C. (2014). Culture of cruelty: Why bullying thrives in higher education, *The Guardian,* November 2014.

21. Tepper, B. J., Duffy, M. K., and Breaux-Soignet, D. M. (2011). Abusive supervision as political activity: Distinguishing impulsive and strategic expressions of downward hostility. In G. Ferris, and D. Treadway (Eds.), *Politics in Organizations,* pp. 191–212 (Routledge Press, USA).

22. Tedeschi, J. T., and Felson, R. B. (1994). Violence, Aggression, and Coercive Actions (American Psychological Association, USA).

23. Kiazad, K., Restubog, S. L. D., Zagenczyk, T. J., Kiewitz, C., and Tang, R. L. (2010). In pursuit of power: The role of authoritarian leadership in the relationship between supervisors' Machiavellianism and subordinates' perceptions of abusive supervisory behavior, *Journal of Research in Personality,* 44, pp. 512–519.

24. Waldman, D. A., Wang, D., Hannah, S. T., Owens, B.P., and Balthazard, P. A. (2017). Psychological and neurological predictors of abusive supervision, *Personnel Psychology,* 71(3), pp. 399–421.

25. Campbell, W. K., Bonacci, A. M., Shelton, J., Exline, J. J., and Bushman, B. J. (2013). Psychological entitlement: Interpersonal consequences and validation of a self-report measure, *Journal of Personality Assessment,* 83, pp. 29–45.

26. Khan, A. K., Moss, S. E., Quratulain, S., and Hameed, I. (2018). When and how subordinate performance leads to abusive supervision: A social dominance perspective, *Journal of Management,* 44, pp. 2801–2826.

27. Burton, J. P., Hoobler, J. M., and Scheuer, M. L. (2012). Supervisor workplace stress and abusive supervision: The buffering effect of exercise, *Journal of Business and Psychology,* 27(3), pp. 271–279.

28. Aryee, S., Chen, Z. X., Sun, L.-Y., and Debrah, Y. A. (2007). Antecedents and outcomes of abusive supervision: Test of a trickle-down model, *Journal of Applied Psychology,* 92(1), pp. 191–201.

29. Rafferty, A. E., Restubog, S. L. D., and Jimmieson, N. L. (2010). Losing sleep: Examining the cascading effects of supervisors' experience of injustice on subordinates' psychological health. *Work and Stress*, 24, pp. 36–55.

30. Tedeschi, J. T., and Norman, N. M. (1985). A social psychological interpretation of displaced aggression, *Advances in Group Processes*, 2, pp. 29–56.

31. Else, H. (2018). Top geneticist loses £3.5-million grant in first test of landmark bullying policy, *Nature*, 560, p. 420.

32. Jordão, E. M. A. (2019). PhDs in Brazil are perishing even when they publish, *Nature Human Behaviour*, 3, p. 1015.

33. Moss, S. E. (2018). Research is set up for bullies to thrive, *Nature*, 500, p. 529.

34. Lavers, J. (2019). Career satisfaction falls prey to bottomless demands, *Nature Human Behaviour*, 3, p. 1020.

35. Kupferschmidt, K. (2018). New case of alleged bullying rocks the Max Planck Society, *Science*, 361(6403), pp. 630–631.

36. Tepper, B. J., Moss, S. E., and Duffy, M. K. (2011). Predictors of abusive supervision: Supervisor perceptions of deep-level dissimilarity, relationship conflict, and subordinate performance, *Academy of Management Journal*, 54, pp. 279–294.

37. Opotow, S. (1990). Moral exclusion and injustice: An introduction, *Journal of Social Issues*, 46(1), pp. 1–20.

38. Elias, R. (1986). *The Politics of Victimization: Victims, Victimology, and Human Rights* (Oxford University Press, United Kingdom).

39. Olweus, D. (1978). *Aggression in Schools: Bullies and Whipping Boys* (Hemisphere Publishing Corporation, USA).

40. Tepper B. J., and Simon, L. S. (2015). Employee maintenance: Examining employment relationships from the perspective of managerial leaders, *Research in Personal and Human Resources Management*, 33, pp. 1–50.

41. Harrison, D. A., and Klein, K. J. (2007). What's the difference? Diversity constructs as separation, variety, or disparity in organizations, *Academy of Management Review*, 32(4), pp. 1199–1228.

42. Hentschel, T., Shemla, M., Wegge, J., and Kearney, E. (2013). Perceived diversity and team functioning: The role of diversity beliefs and affect, *Small Group Research*, 44, pp. 33–61.

43. McMillan, A., Chen, H., Richard, O. C., and Bhuian, S. N. (2012). A mediation model of task conflict in vertical dyads: Linking

organizational culture, subordinate values, and subordinate outcomes, *International Journal of Conflict Management*, 23, pp. 307–332.

44. Woehr, D. J., Arciniega, L. M., and Poling, T. L. (2012). Exploring the effects of value diversity on team effectiveness, *Journal of Business and Psychology*, 28, pp. 107–121.

45. "Science remains male-dominated" (2017). *The Economist*, March 11.

46. "Doctoral degrees earned by women, by major" (2020). *APS Physics*.

47. Mahmoudi, M. (2020). Academic bullying: Desperate for data and solutions, *Science*, January 16.

48. McConnell, S. C., Westerman, E. L., Pierre, J. F., Heckler, E. J., and Schwartz, N. B. (2018). Research: United States national postdoc survey results and the interaction of gender, career choice and mentor impact, *eLife*, 7, e40189.

49. Turban, D. B., and Jones, A. P. (1988). Supervisor-subordinate similarity: Types, effects and mechanisms, *Journal of Applied Psychology*, 73, pp. 228–234.

50. Walter, F., Lam, C. K., ven der Vegt, G. S., Huang, X, and Miao, Q. (2015). Abusive supervision and subordinate performance: Instrumentality considerations in the emergence and consequences of abusive supervision, *Journal of Applied Psychology*, 100, pp. 1056–1072.

51. Sidanius, J., Levin, S., Liu, J., and Pratto, F. (2000). Social dominance orientation, anti-egalitarianism and the political psychology of gender: An extension and cross-cultural replication, *European Journal of Social Psychology*, 30, pp. 41–67.

52. Anonymous (2018). Bullies have no place in academia—even if they're star scientists, *The Guardian*, December, 2017.

53. Fox, S., and Spector, P. E. (2010). Instrumental counterproductive behavior and the theory of planned behavior: A "cold cognitive" approach to complement "hot affective" theories of CWB. In C. A. Schriesheim, and L. L. Neider (Eds.), *Research in Management: The Dark Side of Management*, pp. 93–114 (Information Age, USA).

54. Hobfoll, S. E. (1989). Conservation of resources: A new attempt at conceptualizing stress, *American Psychologist*, 44(3), pp. 513–524.

55. Mahmoudi, M., and Moss, S. (2019). Scarcity of lab positions in high-ranked institutions creates a breeding ground for bullies, *BioImpacts*, 9(4), p. 251.

56. French, J. R. P., Jr., and Raven, B. (1959). The bases of social power. In D. Cartwright (Ed.), *Studies in Social Power*, pp. 150–167 (University of Michigan Press, USA).

57. "Doctorates: PhD gender gap" (2017). Available at: Naturejobs.com, May 24.

58. Flaherty, C. (2017). The prestige gap, Inside Higher Ed, February 8.

59. Nature Editorial Board (2018). Stop exploitation of foreign postdocs in the United States. *Nature*, 563, p. 444.

Chapter 4

Targets' Responses to Abusive Supervision

Sherry Moss
Wake Forest University, USA
mosss@wfu.edu

After writing an Opinion piece for *Nature* in the fall of 2018 on the occurrence of bullying in academic science,[1] I was overwhelmed with email correspondence and phone calls from those who had been targeted or who had observed this phenomenon. The majority of emails I received contained heart-wrenching accounts of tragic stories from PhD students or postdocs who had endured remarkably cruel treatment from their PIs (principal investigators). They also shared their stories on how they responded to the abuse.

To discuss targets' responses to abusive supervision, I will first review the literature from the field of organization behavior on targets' responses to bullying. Then, I will share stories from my correspondence with targets of bullying in academic science and show that their typical responses fall into one of the two categories:

A Brief Guide to Academic Bullying
Edited by Morteza Mahmoudi
Copyright © 2022 Jenny Stanford Publishing Pte. Ltd.
ISBN 978-981-4877-79-4 (Paperback), 978-1-003-16034-2 (eBook)
www.jennystanford.com

(1) "Code of Silence" and (2) "Report the Bully." I will then illuminate the typically disastrous results of both of these choices.

4.1 Research on Coping Behavior

There are several dozen studies in the field of organization behavior that focus on how employees cope with abusive supervision. Coping is defined as the "conscious, volitional attempts to regulate the environment or one's reaction to the environment under stressful conditions."[2] Studies reveal that there are many employee coping strategies, including retaliation and revenge, upward hostility, displaced hostility, problem drinking, withdrawal behavior, turnover, direct confrontation, avoidance, and ingratiation.[3-9] According to a recent review of the literature, due to the disjointed nature of the research, evaluating only two or three coping strategies at a time, there is still a lot to be uncovered before researchers and practitioners can determine which strategies are effective and which ones are not.[10] In the meantime, one may classify the typical responses as aggressive and nonaggressive.

4.1.1 Aggressive Responses

One of the most studied responses to abusive supervision is an aggressive response, primarily retaliation. Mitchell and Ambrose found that employees engaged in three different retaliatory responses following abuse from their supervisors: supervisor-directed deviance, organizational deviance, and interpersonal deviance.[4] Supervisor-directed deviance is a form of retaliation that is intended to "make the supervisor pay" for his or her aggression toward the target. Retaliatory responses range from passive-aggressive (e.g., "refused to talk to my supervisor," "gossiped about my supervisor") to actively aggressive (e.g., "swore at my supervisor," "publicly embarrassed my supervisor"). There is significant evidence to support the notion that employees engage in this type of behavior when they feel that they've been abused.[11] Mitchell and Ambrose[4] found that of the three responses they studied, supervisor-directed deviance was the most likely and this was especially true when the target had strong negative reciprocity beliefs (e.g., "If someone treats you badly, you should treat that person badly in return").[12] In addition, evidence suggests that certain personality characteristics or perceptions moderate the relationship between abusive supervision and supervisor-directed retaliation. A target's lack of self-control or a belief that one's supervisor has little punitive power will increase the likelihood of supervisor-directed aggression in response to abusive supervision.[11]

On the contrary, other studies suggest that when power differentials are high, retaliation is significantly less frequent, likely due to fear of retaliation from the abusive supervisor.[13] In academic science, there is little evidence of overt retaliation toward the supervisor,[14] presumably due to the high stakes of crossing one's PI and risking one's future in science by provoking a punitive response such as a poor recommendation, reputational damage, or revoked funding, all of which are controlled by the senior scientist.[15] This power differential, combined with a perceived lack of mobility to move to another lab/supervisor,[7] creates a situation where one is stuck with the abuse and perceives no good alternatives. One of the individuals who wrote to me about witnessing the abuse of a PhD student validated this observation. In this case, the bully used his coercive powers to extend the student's "sentence" in his lab:

A PhD student in the lab got a job offer when he was 5.5 years into his PhD training. He told our PI that he wished to accept that offer, and the company was willing to wait for eight months for his graduation. Our PI replied instantly: "No, decline it. You are not ready". That student kept working in the lab waiting for graduation. Our school has a time limit for a PhD training, which is 7 + 1, which means the maximum allowance for PhD is 7 years with one year provision if it is really necessary. In his 7th year, our PI told him not to worry, he could write a letter to the dean asking for the 8th. At this point, unfortunately his wife stopped working and the whole family with children lived on his graduate student stipend. They were on government support and his wife did not have health insurance. There was not a subsidy for health care for dependents of graduate students so they were not able to purchase healthcare. In a meeting with our PI, he told him: "I need to graduate so I can find a job to support my family." "No, you are not ready yet, don't you care about your science?" replied our PI. "I only care about feeding my family," replied the graduate student. Everyone in the lab was shocked when we were told about the conversation. Even after that conversation, the graduate student remained trapped. To the end of his 8th year, our PI told him not to worry, he will write another letter to extend. Everyone knows by the 8th year, by strict school's rule, he will not be able to register as a student. He could continue his PhD, but as a volunteer in the lab without pay.

This narrative illustrates why an aggressive response toward the PI supervisor is unlikely. The power differentials and the supervisor control of resources strongly discourage an aggressive response. When employees are unable to direct their retaliation toward their abusive supervisors, they may, instead, displace their hostility toward the organization in general, toward others within the organization (besides the supervisor), or even toward family members.[16] Typical organizational responses include shirking responsibilities, taking longer breaks, stealing office supplies, or reducing effort.[17] Interpersonal deviance involves directing aggressive behaviors at others in the workplace, coworkers, for example (e.g., yelling or cursing at a coworker, publicly embarrassing a coworker, or losing one's temper).[17] Hoobler and Brass found that abused employees were more likely to engage in family undermining (e.g., "my family member often takes negative work emotions out on me"),[16] while Carlson et al. found that the partners of abused employees were more likely to report increased conflict and tension in their relationships than those of non-abused employees.[18] This set of findings indicates that abused employees respond by directing their retaliatory behaviors not only toward the abusive supervisor, but also toward the organization, colleagues, and family members.[4,19] Interestingly, this displaced aggression is very similar to the displaced aggression toward subordinates that abusive supervisors engage in when they lack self-control,[20] are being mistreated by their own supervisors,[21] or pressured from above.[22] While I have seen no specific evidence that targets of abuse in academic science engage in displaced aggression, this trickle-down explanation for supervisors' abuse toward employees and their employees' subsequent displaced aggression toward others is extremely concerning as it helps to explain the toxic culture of abuse that arises in many labs, effectively spreading bullying behavior beyond the supervisor–employee dyad.

4.2 Nonaggressive Responses

Much of the research on coping comes from the literature on workplace stressors. This literature, which supports the idea that abusive supervisors represent a significant source of workplace stress,[23] describes likely coping responses as either active or avoidant.[24] Active (but nonaggressive) strategies are aimed at problem-solving and typically involve direct attempts to address or overcome the stressor. Avoidant strategies are focused on escaping from the stressful situation and avoiding noxious stimuli altogether.[25] Three studies[6,8,25] hypothesized and found that the targets of abusive supervision were more likely to engage in avoidant strategies such as leaving work early, avoiding the supervisor ("avoid delivering bad news to him/her" or "talk only superficially with him/her"), and psychological withdrawal (e.g., "left work as soon as possible," "daydreamed or imagined a better time or place," or "wished the situation would go away"), effectively distancing themselves from their abusers either physically or psychologically.

While utilized less frequently than avoidant strategies, some abused employees engaged in the active strategy of directly, but nonaggressively, addressing the abuser or those who might help (e.g., upper leadership). Examples of this type of active strategy include speaking up when treated unjustly or talking to someone who could do something concrete about the problem.[24] Tepper et al.[8] found that when employees engaged in direct and active coping, they reduced their psychological distress (i.e., anxiety, depression, and emotional exhaustion) and when they engaged in avoidant coping, their psychological distress was greater. Nandkeolyar et al. also found that abused subordinates were more likely to engage in avoidant coping and that their performance was lower when they used avoidant coping strategies than when they used active strategies.[26] This set of findings suggests that abused subordinates have a coping dilemma.[8] The strategy that is more likely to bring them relief and better performance (i.e., active, direct coping) is less likely to be used and the strategy that results in greater distress and lower performance (i.e., avoidant coping) is the more frequently used strategy. If active, direct strategies work to reduce distress, and possibly increase performance, then why don't abused employees use them more?

As discussed above, in the case of academic bullying, the likely explanation is fear of retribution. This concern is illustrated in my correspondence with an abused PhD student:

> I am a PhD Biochemistry student and am experiencing [academic bullying]. However, I have no courage to speak up for myself because of fear that it could affect my status as an International Student. I never talked to more senior faculty members even though I know they would listen and be supportive of me (actually, the department itself is very welcoming and encouraging). I only talk to my lab mates who experience the same things as I do. Right now, I think I still can handle the stress until I graduate in the coming summer. I know it is wrong that I don't speak up but there are times I also need to protect myself. I'm already a 4th year PhD candidate and with just one wrong move, my graduation could be compromised.

An alternative, nonaggressive coping strategy is ingratiation. Ingratiation is defined as an attempt to further one's personal interests through flattery, conformity, or performing favors.[27] With the goal of exerting some social influence and attempting to gain control over a toxic work environment, abused subordinates may engage in ingratiation tactics to reduce the negative effects of abusive supervision. Harvey et al.[9] attempted to determine how ingratiation could impact the relationship between abusive supervision and employee outcomes. They found that ingratiation, especially when paired with positive affect (i.e., displaying enthusiasm), reduced the negative impact of abusive supervision on job tension, emotional exhaustion, and turnover intentions. While this study provides no evidence that ingratiation or the display of positive affect *reduces* abusive supervision, it does provide evidence that flattering or doing favors for the abusive supervisor or behaving in an interested, enthusiastic, and attentive manner toward the abuser can be effective in attenuating the negative consequences of abuse.

The last set of nonaggressive responses to abusive supervision can best be described as palliative or escape behaviors. In studies of medical students and interns, abusive supervision was shown to be directly associated with problem drinking.[28] Bamberger and Bacharach[5] found a direct, positive relationship between abusive supervision and problem drinking (e.g., had a drink first thing in the morning or felt annoyed by others criticizing your drinking), suggesting that abused employees use alcohol as a palliative response or as an escape from their reality. Another form of escape is psychological withdrawal, defined as psychologically distancing oneself from a stressful situation such as an abusive supervisor.[29] Psychological withdrawal provides a mental escape from work and might include behaviors such as cyberloafing, working on personal matters at work, or shirking work responsibilities.[30] These behaviors not only serve as an escape but could also be considered forms of retaliation against the organizational as discussed above.[17] Of course, the ultimate form of withdrawal behavior is leaving the organization, but this is most likely when employees perceive there are alternative sources of employment,[7] which is a key to understanding why abused graduate students and postdocs do not leave their labs or their PIs.

4.3 Responses to Bullying in Academic Science

4.3.1 Code of Silence

As discussed above, it is very difficult for bullied employees to respond aggressively or even to directly confront an abusive supervisor due to the fear of retaliation. Among the many targets with whom I've corresponded, there is a "code of silence" that is real and palpable. It is consistent with the amount of coercive power PIs hold over their students, postdocs, and junior colleagues and resembles the avoidant coping strategies discussed above, which are more likely to be used when the target feels there are few alternative options to change labs, where there are significant power differentials, and when there is fear of retribution. These sentiments are summed up by one of the targets who reached out to me:

> I work as a Post-Doctoral fellow and am about to complete my first year. After reading your article I felt it was like my story too. I am also constantly facing yelling on small things, discouraging comments, comments about personal life, etc. by my PI. I tried to figure out if there is any solution or not and the conclusion is, I can't do anything except search for a new lab. I learned from someone that if your PI has funding then the administration will try to avoid taking any steps against him. Also, my PI has all the rights to deport me and my family

from US within 24 hours, because everything for me depends upon his recommendations or approval. Like me, there will be many suffering regularly, then what is the remedy for such things? Be prepared to leave your career midway whenever your PI wants or just tolerate everything?

—Postdoc fellow, Cancer Research

The code of silence often extends beyond the target's time in the toxic lab. Once the target leaves the lab, there are further incentives not to report the bully. Reputation in the field is a key motivator, along with a feeling of powerlessness, which is at least partially attributable to the significant psychological damage caused by the bully:

I too experienced this, along with an entire lab of 20 others. It was mostly verbal and psychological abuse and it was extensive. The problem was that the PI brought in a lot of grant money and so the universities would do nothing about it. Secondly, as you mentioned, one risks losing years of work as well as being damaged by verbal comments and recommendations letters. These letters are particularly problematic as they are considered confidential. I had a girlfriend at the time who was a clinical psychologist and she told me this PI was basically a psychopath. They referred to them as CEO psychopaths. It took me a while to understand this as it is difficult for the target to see clearly sometimes, especially early on. However, this was spot on. The damage was considerable and lasting. I still have bad dreams about it. I am considering doing something about it now but I'm not sure what, other than alert the appropriate parties. I'm still in the same field but I'm not sure my stature is secure enough to go after this. However, as with the "me too" movement, the only way to combat this problem is to expose the perpetrators and the extensive university network of deans and presidents that protect them.

The "code of silence" includes the use of avoidant tactics as well as refraining from reporting abusive behaviors to the institution. One study showed that only 2% of targets will report the bullying.[31] Let us now try to understand why targets do not report the abuse. Reasons include the absence of legal and institutional protocols for bullying, the resulting unwillingness of institutions to act, and the power and importance of prolific, grant-getting scientists whom institutions do not wish to lose as illustrated in the narratives above.

4.3.2 Reporting of Abuse and Institutional Silence

While much of the evidence supports the code of silence strategy for dealing with bullies, there is some evidence that targets will report the abuse to officials such as human resources (HR) departments, department chairs, deans, or upper administration.[14] Unfortunately, all too often, institutional responses are minimal and deficient. In the first case reported below, HR did nothing to address this target's concerns.

> Before leaving my last job at XXX, I tried to approach the HR & Diversity and Inclusion Department for a solution, but they could not do anything. According to them, if they notice a 'repeated pattern in the behavior of my supervisor, then this is an issue to be pursued' but not if the concerns are raised by only 1 or 2 persons from a lab. Although I was the second one to approach them to point out my concern, nothing changed, and I planned to leave ultimately.
>
> —Postdoctoral Fellow, Cancer Research

Two reasons for the lack of response from institutions are (1) the conscious decision to protect their best scientists and (2) the absence of institutional and legal protocols for addressing bullying. Unlike sexual harassment, which has clear legal guidelines to follow for those receiving reports from targets, bullying has no such protocols, legal or institutional.[32] Both of these motivations are illustrated in the two narratives below:

> I am a postdoc fellow for 3 years now, and I would like to share some thoughts with you. Apart from the obvious shouting or violent behavior that some PIs might have, there are other less visible ways of bullying that I experienced and no one talks about—or at least didn't find it yet. Sometimes it's less obvious, but some professors that are so well supported and covered by the universities, act in a way that has terrible consequences for their PhD students and post-docs. They are so selfish about their careers, that they are capable of doing whatever they could to take advantage and advance in their own careers at the expense of the most vulnerable ones. As a consequence they block all kind of opportunities for post-docs, ignore them, and give benefits only to the favorite ones. For some years I suffered a lot by working in a toxic environment like this. Unfortunately, it could get extremely difficult to find another position and quit. And the worst part is that at

the end, apart from being depressed, your self-esteem has decreased considerably, you realize you lost years of your life/academic career, and you are completely alone, without any kind of support or mentorship. In addition, the professor is still enjoying their powerful status, and of course Universities don't do anything, they just look to other side as nothing happened, because usually these predator professors are the ones bringing money to the University, so they will never punish them because they want to keep them. Making the decision to leave from a context like this is extremely hard, especially because young scholars rely heavily and depend on their supervisors and previous bosses writing good recommendation letters in order to get a new job. But many times these professors don't want to be abandoned [by their students so] they write bad letters or punish the young scholar whenever they have the chance. Sometimes it looks like only sexual harassment situations are serious enough to act and make justice. But what happens when the one committing these acts is a woman and there are no sexual issues involved? I think it is important that we pay attention to these situations too.

—Female Postdoc

I had a very traumatic time at one of the first class institutions after making allegations against my supervisor for professional misconduct (abusive behavior and research misconduct). I was a postdoc who developed a novel protocol which represented big progress in my field of study and I was awarded a 2 year fellowship grant to support my research. I was preparing my manuscript for *Nature* journal but my supervisor manipulated some of the data intentionally to increase the chance of publication and despite my efforts asking him for correction and clarification of his wrong deeds, he submitted the paper to *Nature*. I again asked him to fix this but he was bullying me, and forcing me as always and pressuring me to be ok with whatever he wanted to do. This was not the first time he had forced me to participate in research misconduct and I refused to do so. Once I asked him again he outburst his anger over me and showed me a violent response banging on his desk and yelling. He told me "I did this for you." I was scared a lot and thought next time he will hit me so I went and reported him to the director of the department. I didn't know this could be the beginning of an endless nightmare for me. I have gone through a lot including so many humiliations, threats, intimidations, retaliations, discriminations, harassments etc., all publicly! They tried their best to ruin my reputation, and all other opportunities to stay in the same field and withheld my paper from publication, revoked my grant and my visa! They ruined my mental health, life and entire career to save their reputation. Although based on school rules and federal laws, I should not be subjected to such adverse actions and my reputation and position should be protected by the institution.

—Female Medical Postdoc

This foreign postdoc went on to be blackballed, was unable to find another position easily, and was working as a cleaning lady when I spoke to her on the phone.

It is clear that there are at least two important motivations driving institutions' absence of acceptable action following allegations of abuse. First, they do not have legal protocols to follow. This, combined with the desire to retain prolific researchers and grant receivers, typically causes targets who report abuse to be in worse shape than when they were silent. Despite these motivations not to act on reports of academic bullying, some institutional attempts to understand the bullying problem backfire, leaving victims the targets of additional abuse:

It happened that for an untold reason, our department sent a questionnaire survey to lab members asking for our evaluation of our principal of investigator (PI), aka advisor. Some filled it in as a formality thinking it will not change anything, while the others wrote their opinion. Although the survey was said to be anonymous, our PI was allowed to read them all, seeing two out of seven are bad evaluations. During a lab meeting, in front of everyone, he made a statement: "I can't believe you could say bad things about me to others. I request that you not to say anything bad about me to any outside people. I always try to write good recommendations for you when asked, but if I write my honest opinion about all of you, none of you can ever find a job." That was said as a threat. He never asked us what was wrong, and how could things be fixed.

Overall, the research from organizational behavior and academic science, along with these narratives, presents a grim reality for those suffering from abusive supervision. First, we do not know which coping strategies result in the best outcomes. We only know which ones make targets feel better. Evidence from academic science is consistent with the research from organizational behavior—doing nothing is a common strategy and it results in continued misery. Finding support from friends, colleagues, and family appears to be the safest and most likely response.[14] For those rare few who choose to report the abuse, anecdotal evidence and research reports suggest that it is rare for targets to find relief from their organizations.[14] For these reasons, it is ever more critical for the larger field of academic science to take a systematic and comprehensive approach to addressing this problem.[32]

References

1. Moss, S.E. (2018). Research is set up for bullies to thrive. *Nature*, 500, p. 529.

2. Connor-Smith, J.K., and Flachsbart, C. (2007). Relations between personality and coping: A meta-analysis. *Journal of Personality and Social Psychology*, 93(6), pp. 1080–1107.

3. Aquino, K., Tripp, T.M., and Bies, R.J. (2001). How employees respond to personal offense: The effects of blame attribution, victim status, and offender status on revenge and reconciliation in the workplace. *Journal of Applied Psychology*, 86(1), pp. 52–59.

4. Mitchell, M.S., and Ambrose, M.L. (2007). Abusive supervision and workplace deviance and the moderating effects of negative reciprocity beliefs. *Journal of Applied Psychology*, 92(4), pp. 1159–1168.

5. Bamberger, P.A., and Bacharach, S.B. (2006). Abusive supervision and subordinate problem drinking: Taking resistance, stress and subordinate personality into account. *Human Relations*, 59(6), pp. 723–752.

6. Mawritz, M.B., Dust, S.B., and Resick, C.J. (2014). Hostile climate, abusive supervision, and employee coping: Does conscientiousness matter? *Journal of Applied Psychology*, 99(4), pp. 737–747.

7. Tepper, B.J. (2000). Consequences of abusive supervision. *Academy of Management Journal*, 43(2), pp. 178–190.

8. Tepper, B.J., Moss, S.E., Lockhart, D.E., and Carr, J.C. (2007). Abusive supervision, upward maintenance communication, and subordinates' psychological distress. *Academy of Management Journal*, 50, pp. 1160–1180.

9. Harvey, P., Stoner, J., Hochwarter, W., and Kacmar, C. (2007). Coping with abusive supervision: The neutralizing effects of

ingratiation and positive effect on negative employee outcomes. *The Leadership Quarterly*, 18(3), pp. 264–280.

10. Tepper, B.J., Simon, L., and Park, H.M. (2017). Abusive supervision. *Annual Review of Organizational Psychology and Organizational Behavior*, 4, pp. 123–152.

11. Lian, H., Brown, D.J., Ferris, D.L., Liang, L.H., Keeping, L.M., and Morrison, R. (2014). Abusive supervision and retaliation: A self-control framework. *Academy of Management Journal*, 57(1), pp. 116–139.

12. Eisenberger, R., Lynch, P., Aselage, J., and Rohdieck, S. (2004). Who takes the most revenge? Individual differences in negative reciprocity norm endorsement. *Personality and Social Psychology Bulletin*, 30(6), pp. 789–799.

13. Aquino, K., Tripp, T.M., and Bies, R.J. (2006). Getting even or moving on? Power, procedural justice, and types of offense as predictors of revenge, forgiveness, reconciliation, and avoidance in organizations. *Journal of Applied Psychology*, 91(3), pp. 653–668.

14. Keashly, L. (2019). Workplace Bullying, Mobbing and Harassment in Academe: Faculty Experience. In: D'Cruz P., Noronha E., Keashly L., and Tye-Williams S. (eds) Special topics and particular occupations, professions and sectors. *Handbooks of Workplace Bullying, Emotional Abuse and Harassment*, vol 4. Springer, Singapore. https://doi. org/10.1007/978-981-10-5154-8_13-1

15. Anonymous (2018). Bullies have no place in academia—even if they're star scientists. *The Guardian*, December 2018.

16. Hoobler, J.M., and Brass, D.J. (2006). Abusive supervision and family undermining as displaced aggression. *Journal of Applied Psychology*, 91(5), pp. 1125–1133.

17. Bennett, R.J., and Robinson, S.L. (2000). Development of a measure of workplace deviance. *Journal of Applied Psychology*, 85(3), pp. 349–360.

18. Carlson, D.S., Ferguson, M., Perrewe, P.L., and Whitten, D. (2011). The fallout from abusive supervision: An examination of subordinates and their partners. *Personnel Psychology*, 64(4), pp. 937–961.

19. Tepper, B.J., and Almeda, M. (2012). Negative Exchanges with Supervisors. In: Eby L. and Allen T. (eds) *Personal Relationships at Work: The Effect of Supervisory, Co-Worker, Team and Customer and Nonwork Exchanges on Employee Attitudes, Behavior, and Well-Being*, pp. 67–93. Routledge Press, USA.

20. Zhang, Y., and Bednall, T.C. (2016). Antecedents of abusive supervision: A meta-analytic review. *Journal of Business Ethics*, 139, pp. 455–471.

21. Mawritz, M.B., Mayer, D.M., Hoobler, J.M., Wayne, S.J., and Marinova, S.V. (2012). A trickle-down model of abusive supervision. *Personnel Psychology*, 65, pp. 325–357.

22. Burton, J.P., Hoobler, J.M., and Scheuer, M.L. (2012). Supervisor workplace stress and abusive supervision: The buffering effect of exercise. *Journal of Business and Psychology*, 27(3), pp. 271–279.

23. Aquino, K., and Thau, S. (2009). Workplace victimization: Aggression from the target's perspective. *Annual Review of Psychology*, 60, pp. 717–741.

24. Lazarus, R.S., and Folkman, S. (1984). *Stress, Appraisal, and Coping* (Springer, USA).

25. Rachlin, H. (1976). *Behavior and Learning* (W. H. Freeman, USA).

26. Nandkeolyar, A.K., Shaffer, J.A., Li, A., Ekkirala, S., and Bagger, J. (2014). Surviving an abusive supervisor: The joint roles of conscientiousness and coping strategies. *Journal of Applied Psychology*, 99(1), pp. 138–150.

27. Tedeschi, J.T., and Melburg, V. (1984). Impression Management and Influence in the Organization. In: Bacharach S.B. and Lawler E.J. (eds) *Research in the Sociology of Organizations*, pp. 31–58. JAI, USA.

28. Richman, J.A., Flaherty, J.A., and Pyskoty, C. (1992). Shifts in problem drinking during a life transition: Adaptation to medical school training. *Journal of Studies on Alcohol*, 53(1), pp. 17–24.

29. Hanisch, K.A., and Hulin, C.L. (1991). General attitudes and organizational withdrawal: An evaluation of a causal model. *Journal of Vocational Behavior*, 39(1), pp. 110–128

30. Tepper, B.J., Duffy, M.K., and Shaw, J.D. (2001). Personality moderators of the relationship between abusive supervision and subordinates' resistance. *Journal of Applied Psychology*, 86(5), pp. 974–983.

31. Zabrodska, K., and Kveton, P. (2013). Prevalence and forms of workplace bullying among university employees. *Employee Responsibilities and Rights Journal*, 25(2), pp. 89–108.

32. Mahmoudi, M. (2020). Academic bullying: Desperate for data and solutions, *Science*, Jan. 16, 2020.

Chapter 5

Mobbing in Academia

Mehdi Kamali,[a] Saman Hosseinpour,[b] Jennifer Swann,[c] Hossein Pooya Sareh,[d] and Morteza Mahmoudi[a]

[a]*Michigan State University, USA*
[b]*University of Erlangen-Nuremberg, Germany*
[c]*Lehigh University, Pennsylvania, USA*
[d]*University of Liverpool, England*
mahmou22@msu.edu

The word "mob" is defined in the Merriam-Webster dictionary as "to crowd around or into noisily, as from curiosity or hostility."[1] The present participle of "mob," "mobbing," is a complicated term. Similar to, for example, nuclear energy, which could be used for peaceful purposes and advancements, such as electricity production and medical applications, or could be applied in destructive ways to produce nuclear bombs for mass destruction, "mobbing" can be utilized constructively and destructively, depending on its use and the domain of application. In this chapter, we explain mobbing in academia as a backdoor retaliation strategy for bullies to pressure targets to withdraw their complains and/or to make biased and usually falsified allegations against targets to put them in corner.

A Brief Guide to Academic Bullying
Edited by Morteza Mahmoudi
Copyright © 2022 Jenny Stanford Publishing Pte. Ltd.
ISBN 978-981-4877-79-4 (Paperback), 978-1-003-16034-2 (eBook)
www.jennystanford.com

5.1   Types of Mobbing

Historically, the origin of mobbing among humans is attributed to the Darwinian struggle for survival by Konrad Lorenz.[2] He observed similar behaviors among birds and other animals and believed that humans adapted the innate impulse via evolution with an excellent ability of rational control.

In programing, developing a software through inclusion of the entire team at the same space, time, computer, and code is referred to as "mob programming" (sometimes "pair programming"), which is known as a positive mobbing action. In this application, all collaborating team members use a single computer to add or remove their codes.[3] Similarly, in another form of positive mobbing which is observed in antipredator adaptation in animals' behavior, the targeted preys gather a team of individuals from similar species to protect their offspring by different actions, such as seducing, harassing, or attacking predators.[4] Antipredator adaptation is mainly observed in birds; however, other animals such as bovines and meerkats also show similar mannerisms. Mobbing behaviors in animals are usually triggered by a "mobbing call," which is a signal among individuals of similar species to unite and prepare for an opportunity to attack the predator.[3,5]

In contrast to the abovementioned examples, mobbing is often defined as a negative behavior. For instance, the law of Scotland defines mobbing as "engaging in a disorderly and criminal behavior, which is usually accompanied by rioting, which may lead to violence or intimidation."[6] In sociological terms, mobbing in the context of human bullying behavior has an extended definition and could include groups of people such as members of a family, school, or workplace as well as communities that align with the bullying process. Within this definition, a person may be mobbed or bullied in the workplace by a group composed of coworkers or associates ranked at higher levels "ganging up" on a target. The ultimate goal of this type of mobbing is often to isolate and force the target to leave the workplace. Hence, the mobbing group may use a variety or combination of methods, which include physical and mental manipulations to disgrace the target via humiliation, intimidation, spreading rumors, discrediting, and innuendo behaviors. Nevertheless, in this definition, mobbing does not refer to sexual or racial harassment.[7]

5.2 Academic Mobbing

The academic environment is an excellent example in which mobbing exists in many different levels. Westhues definition of "mobbing" as "an impassioned, collective campaign by co-workers to exclude, punish, and humiliate a targeted worker"[2] depicts well the action of bullies in academia. This definition has earned international attention and become a common expression describing "academic mobbing." Owing to the nature of power differences, educational institutions such as colleges and universities among various organizations exhibit higher instances of mobbing.[8] In fact, mobbing is being considered as organizational "norms" which may encourage such behaviors.[9]

In conjunction with the other forms of workplace bullying in academia, discussed in other chapters, academic mobbing is considered as one of the toughest and most complex types of bullying. In this regard, the targeted victim is confronted through a combination of different harmful methods such as harassment, humiliation, unjustified accusations, intimidation, and isolation. Unfortunately, this kind of behavior is often invisible to others and therefore hard to prove if a complaint is filed.

5.3 Signs of Academic Mobbing

Mobbing in academia develops in three distinct stages, all of which exhibit distinct signs. In each stage, different oppressive and aggressive tactics and activities are utilized to undermine the target. One should consider the fact that these signs may appear in part or as a whole for a target and could also be tactically applied differently due to the possible complex situations of the organization.[3,7,9]

The first stage in academic mobbing begins with "indirect" negative communications among coworkers, other than the targeted individual, and therefore the target is unaware of the situation. Spreading rumors and lies, complaining about action/inaction, mocking frequently, bypassing looks, insinuating in conversations, belittling comments, discrediting the achievements and endeavors of the target, meeting secretly, misinterpreting facts, and supervising rigorously are part of the indirect negative communication stage. All the mentioned adverse actions are utilized in the work and personal life of the target to gather pieces of evidence for later justifications.[7,9]

In the second stage of mobbing, "direct" negative communication begins to form with the aim of blatant and direct confrontation with the target. Sending offensive messages, concealing information, manipulating data, accusing without rational justification, insulting someone for making mistakes, arranging meetings for disciplinary issues, advertising the target as a mentally destabilized person, public humiliation, intimidation, mocking via offering help for a better adaptation, and messing with the target's work area are typically included in the direct negative communication step. The combination of such communications at this stage conveys the message to everyone in the organization that the target is a person who ignores advice, creates problems, has secluded personality and refuses to accept the cultural diversity of the organization, destructs the community through social and mentally adverse behaviors, works individually and not as a team member and meanwhile depends heavily on others due to asking numerous questions, and in general presents a difficult character.

In the third stage, a poisonous atmosphere appears to form among the entire department or the organization via negative communication. As the toxic clouds extend over time by the "mobbers," they will attract more attention from other members on their side. In this case, if the new members are aggressively involved in the mobbing process, they are called "active" mobbers. In contrast, those who ignore the toxic mobbing atmosphere and pretend nothing happened are referred to as so-called "passive" mobbers. In this situation, finding the truth seems to be very difficult since the ambience is already contaminated. Consequently, the majority of exposed members may join the mobbing campaign without any actual knowledge of the target as a result of the presence of the poisonous conditions and the bizarre peer pressure. Hence, the magnification of negative communication among members intensifies the harsh condition, the target is inevitably accused of being a threat to the organization, and eventually it would be a mistake to continue working with him/her.

Brutal tactics and aggressive activities along with negative communication are powerful weapons at all the three stages to destroy and undermine the target's works and endeavors. Some of these systematic tactics and activities are as follows: (1) preventing the target from having a voice in the organization, (2) assembling illegal, fake, fabricated, and planted evidences from the target's personal and working lives, (3) removing the target from the list of invitations for meetings and promotional situations, (4) criticizing or ignoring the target's accomplishments, (5) negatively affecting the sections responsible for promotion of the target to deny his/her promotions, (6) assigning the duties beyond target's abilities to complete, (7) avoiding the target from effectively finishing the normal work duties through the formation of consecutive obstacles, and (8) illegitimately depriving the target of the rights and benefits applied to the other members of the organization.

5.4 Intensity of Academic Mobbing

The academic environment can be very different from other places of employment, such as for-profit companies or government agencies. In the public's perception, highly educated people often work in academia with a focus on rational pioneer subjects. Moreover, academics are responsible of educating the next generation for hopefully an improved future. Thus, the academic environment is expected to offer many flexibilities to support each individual's growth in various perspectives, such as independence and intelligence with mutual respect. Nevertheless, revealing the truth behind the brutality of mobbing in academic environment will shock the academia.

The highly prevailed examples, deeply established violations, regularly reported incidents, and acquiring acceptance as a work method among the faculty members demonstrate the intensity of academic mobbing. In this regard, the target is irrationally convicted at first and the shreds of evidence are fabricated later to justify the conviction, which resembles the show trial of the Stalin's Moscow Trials.[2b,9,10]

The extent of target's vulnerability against intense academic mobbing varies based on a variety of factors, such as personal differences (i.e., ethnicity, sexuality, and skin color), being a local or a foreigner, financial status, the field of study/work, or aggressiveness of a supervisor/manager. Envy of excellence, various heresies (such as scientific, political, or even religious beliefs), and politics of campus are the other factors affecting one's vulnerability against academic mobbing.[11]

The unfortunate outcomes of an intense academic mobbing can include: (1) dismissing the person from the university via denying his/her tenure, (2) early retirement, (3) repeated sick leaves, (4) sudden resignation, (5) withdrawal from major responsibilities, and (6) increase in turnover of employees.[9,12]

5.5   Reasons and Actions Behind Academic Mobbing

Academic mobbing occurs at different levels and its extent varies from personal level to university level and beyond that. There are various reasons behind mobbing in each level and the severity of the mobbing action often results in its escalation toward wider exposure. The conditions that ignite the process of "mobbing" by a group of "troublemakers" against a target include personal motivations, departmental impulses, and campus-wide reasons. Uncivilized mobbing behaviors such as slander, shunning, isolation, and finally elimination are usually enforced on the personal level by tenured faculty members or more powerful individuals because they have additional security.[9,10,13] The deep-down reason in the minds of mobbers could be that the target does not effectively align with and/or does not support their interests and therefore opposes their "culture and values." A variety of explanations could be enclosed by this concept.

On a personal level, the reasons behind academic mobbing could include: (1) earning more money than them, (2) the targets behave differently and the mobbers may not like,[14] (3) the mobber envies the excellence in teaching, research accomplishments, and grant acquisitions by the target,[14] (4) retaliating on a disagreement with a member who promotes later to a higher position such as dean or chair, (5) exercising the influence of power for the sake of achieving higher authority or self-satisfaction to accumulate power through mobbing others, and (6) satisfying the other hidden psychological desires by mobbers to control people.[7]

On a departmental level, relations within the department could deteriorate and eventually convert to mobbing action for reasons such as: (1) challenging the routine departmental practices that mobbers are habituated to,[14] (2) opposing to share the departmental views,[9] and (3) resisting to participate in the group (i.e., gang).[2b,9,10]

When it reaches the campus level, the accusations strategically receive more attention than that in the personal or departmental level. At this level, the news can be disclosed to the media and consequently affect the reputation of the entire campus/university. Reasons behind such serious cases of academic mobbing could be as follows[9,10,12,13]: (1) defending an already deported person from campus due to their policies, (2) obtaining information from serious misconducted actions by influential colleagues, (3) reporting the information from wrongdoing to authorities as a faithfulness action, and (4) criticizing the organization rationally via his or her political heresy in public.

On the departmental and campus levels, one of the major disappointments in the mobbing process is that the university administrations and department of human resources (HR) are either actively or passively involved in the mobbing campaigns to protect the department and campus reputation instead of implementing corrective action. Therefore, that leaves the target without a voice to call out injustices within the organization and very little hope for corrective action. Indeed, such a situation can horrendously affect the physical and mental health of targets,[2b,9,10] which will be discussed in the next section.

In relatively fewer cases, as compared to the mobbing action in the abovementioned levels, authorities outside academic environment (e.g., police, law enforcement organizations, or official judiciary system) might get involved in resolving the problematic situation. Such external organization often perceive the cases of academic mobbing as "minor" and not very serious cases and interpret them as "internal affairs" of the academic institutions, except the cases in which sexual harassment or serious life threats are in question.

5.6 Health Effects

The consequences of mobbing techniques and strategies are so severe that mobbing is categorized as a major public health issue since it may result in negative mental and physical health effects. Therefore, the existence of mobbing in any organization is recognized as a significant organizational deficiency that requires special attention and immediate actions. Some even believe that universities are more destructive places than the other work environments because they advertise building up members and personal growth, yet have a toxic academic institution.[9,15]

As the mobbing process continues over time, the target gradually becomes excluded from the entire organizational contributions, authority, fame, and respect, and his/her academic achievements and influences are revoked. This situation closely resembles the behavior of oppressive governments in which any effort to defend yourself can and will be used against you. In such systems, the victims of violence will be accused incorrectly and then the verdict goes against them. The severity of the mental effects and the extent of pressure in such systematic mobbing actions are so extreme that even if in rare cases mobbers are not able to physically expel the target from the organization, the targets exclude themselves mentally. The targets become less active in their organization and, for instance, lose the courage of applying for grants, extension of projects, hiring new students, and minimize their interactions with their peers and seclude themselves from extracurricular activities. In the more severe cases, the targets tend to resign or pull out of their careers and responsibilities and therefore conduce their own permanent social exclusion. Consequently, tolerating such a severe social isolation may lead to poor mental health, long-term lasting effects, and possibly even suicide.

An unbelievable number of suicides (i.e., estimated about 12%) among mobbed professors indicates the horrendous situation created by mobbers. In the aftermath of Prof. Will Moore's suicide, professor of political science at Arizona State University, the stigma with regard to the mental health in the faculty community was discussed, despite the lack of substantial research showing the higher rate of suicides among academics as compared to the other groups of workers.[16]

An outrageous example of academic mobbing occurred in Canada in 1994, during which a neurologist professor named Justine Sergent at McGill University committed suicide with her husband in their garage with carbon monoxide (CO) gas after two-year exposure to a mobbing campaign from her workplace. She was accused in the mobbing campaign of ethical violations in research procedures.[9,17]

As shown in this infamous example, mobbing can even have detrimental influences on the other family members of the targets who are not even involved in the workplace. The mobbers may believe that the "punishment" is exclusively directed on the target but have no perception of what dreadful peer pressure they are exerting on not only the target but also on the closest individuals around the targets. Enduring depression, anger, mental and physical sickness, and divorce are the common indirect issues formed by mobbers on the targets' innocent family members. In another example, Dr. Janice Harper from the University of Tennessee Knoxville (UTK) in the cultural anthropology program was subjected to academic mobbing in 2007. Even though the situation pushed her toward suicidal thoughts, she eventually managed the situation and found help with her situation. Nevertheless, her daughter went through major trauma in this period and struggled for recovery after the situation resolved.[18]

As a result of academic mobbing, suffering from mental issues such as high stress, anxiety, depression, and occasionally suicidal thoughts is inevitable for victims. Moreover, post-traumatic stress disorder (PTSD) is often reported after exposure to such conditions.[9,15,18] However, policies adopted in many educational institutions to confront mobbing and workplace bullying often appear relatively ineffective due to a variety of protocols developed in every campus and department.[17–19]

5.7 Any Practical Remedy?

The pressure of punishment on the target of a mobbing campaign can never be fully understood by individuals unless they have been previously subjected to the mobbing process. Therefore, the penalty is primarily immoral. The researchers showed that each mobbed person experienced similar predictable patterns and pathways.[9,10,18] Knowing some general useful alleviation steps will assist the academics to mitigate the mobbing effects. Some of these steps are briefly discussed next.

5.7.1 Acquaintance

All academic members need to be aware of the fact that bullying and mobbing are typically endemic across many campuses. It should be openly discussed and shared that the targets of academic mobbing are often severely hurt, physically and mentally. Familiarity with the campaign and the process of academic mobbing can help the academic members to rationally encounter the situation without being shocked or surprised. Especially knowing the steps during which the academic mobbing develops will assist the targets to understand where they are and how to strategically deal with the situation to either prevent further actions or mitigate the damages. Therefore, a certain level of awareness is essential for the whole academic members via workshops, training sessions, regular meetings around the subjects of academic mobbing and academic bullying, and by providing mental health support through compartmentalized campus counseling and wellness services. Moreover, creating a culture of access and inclusion by providing the victims of academic mobbing with the necessary tools and means of coping with the mental and social damages is an effective means to improve the academic climate, especially for the more vulnerable groups of academics.

5.7.2 Vigilance

Vigilance about the indisputable signs and incidents of academic mobbing in departments/campuses is as important as understanding the mobbing process. When an individual witnesses an instigation of a new mobbing campaign through a negative opinion or even a general comment, especially on a colleague, staying vigilant and skeptical is essential for preventing further negative actions and processes. As was mentioned earlier, "passive" mobbers are often part of the mobbing campaigns. It should be emphasized that "passive" mobbers, though unintentionally, indeed partake in an action which sets the precedent for the more systematic mobbing behavior in the future. Such cycle even increases the chance of the "passive" mobbers in the past to become the targets of the mobbing campaigns in the future.

5.7.3 Communication

As the adverse activities such as elimination strategies and initial attempts for recruitments of the "mobbing gang" in an academic mobbing campaign begin to form, the academic peers must raise the red flag immediately and begin to actively participate in the communication about the issue. We always need to keep in mind that horrendous academic mobbing campaigns heavily isolate their targets in a way that disables the individuals to perform their normal activities. Therefore, the targets may not be able to focus on rights or defend themselves even if the laws are already well defined in their favor and to their support. In this situation, we need to reject silence treatment and passive observations. "Nothing strengthens authority as much as silence."— Leonardo da Vinci. "All that is necessary for evil to succeed is that good men/women do nothing."—Winston Churchill.

5.7.4 Resilience and Resistance

The last step in mitigating the academic mobbing effects is resistance against mobbing behaviors along with resilience in the face of mobbing campaigns. It should be emphasized that the process of academic mobbing is complicated and simultaneously needs endurance and flexibility. The active members of the mobbing group think that their actions are ethical and their behavior is best for not only the department but also for the target. Therefore, they forcefully pursue the academic mobbing process to achieve their goals resulting in the expelling or isolating the target. The culture of academic mobbing is a form of tyranny and hence tremendous energy is required for changing the direction of the academic mobbing process.

5.8 Fallacy Behind Academic Mobbing

5.8.1 Academic Mobbing Based on the Mob Appeal Fallacy

In logic and argumentation theory, an *argumentum ad populum* (Latin for "appeal to the people"), also known as "common belief fallacy" and "mob appeal fallacy," is a fallacious argument which claims that a proposition or conclusion must be true because many or a majority of people consider them to be true.[20-24]

Based on one or more mob appeal fallacies, in academic mobbing, a group of academics form a mob to achieve an often predetermined conclusion about the target of mobbing. Generally, the "leaders" of the mob provide their colleagues—hereafter called "followers"—with some biased information about the target, pursuing them—either directly or indirectly—to support an agenda, though the background information of the followers about the target might be negligible to none. As a result of hierarchies and relationships in the institution, the followers often *close ranks* with the leaders opportunistically, as they generally have more interest to support the more powerful side, "politically," and potentially for personal interests such as promotions. Consequently, the target would need to defend against a unified team of bullies.

5.8.2 *A Hundred Authors Against Einstein*: A Historically Significant Case

A significant and documented historical example of such mobbing behavior was against Albert Einstein by the so called "anti-relativists." In particular, a booklet entitled *A Hundred Authors Against Einstein* was published in 1931 with a collection of 28 statements against Einstein's theories of relativity, with an additional group of 92 authors introduced by the editors as Einstein's "further opponents or authors of opposing publications."[25-27]

It was interesting that—according to the investigation by Hubert Goenner[26]—none of the three editors of the booklet were active scientists. However, surprisingly, two of the 28 contributors to the booklet were internationally recognized academics: the philosopher Hans Driesch (1867–1941) and the mathematician Hjalmar Mellin (1854–1933), known for proposing an integral transform known as the Mellin transform. Among them were also the theoretical physicist Jean-Marie Le Roux and the mathematician and World Chess Champion Emanuel Lasker. It is important to notice that while that action was initiated by a small group of individuals, that is, three nonacademics, many academics joined them to support their agenda.

The actions of the contributors to the booklet is a typical example of mobbing through a mob appeal fallacy. In response to publication of the booklet, Einstein wrote a paper entitled "My Response. On the Anti-Relativity Theoretical Co., Ltd.," which started with the following statement:[27,28]

> A motley group has joined together to form a company under the pretentious name "Syndicate of German Scientists" currently with the single purpose of denigrating the theory of relativity and me as its author in the eyes of nonphysicists. Recently Messrs. Weyland and Gehrke held a lecture with this intent at Philharmonic Hall which I attended personally. I am fully aware of the fact that both speakers are unworthy of a reply from my pen; for, I have good reason to believe that there are other motives behind this undertaking than the search for truth. (Were I a German national, whether bearing a swastika or not, rather than a Jew of liberal international bent ...) I only respond because I have received repeated requests from well-meaning quarters to have my view made known.

In fact, the leaders of the campaign against Einstein had supposed that by forming a large team of opponents with different backgrounds they could have formed a strong "mob" to legitimize their opposition. Einstein's response—as given above—implies that he was well aware of the mobbing nature of the booklet and the mob appeal fallacy behind their reasoning. It is well-known that in reaction to the publication of the booklet, Einstein said:[29] "if I were wrong, then one author would have been enough."

References

1. Merriam-Webster, *Definition of mob.* Since 1828.
2. (a) K. Lorenz, et al., *On Aggression.* 1966: Harcourt, Brace & World.

   (b) K. Westhues, *Mobbing, a Natural Fact,* Adapted and revised from *Mobbing am akademischen Arbeitsplatz, a lecture given in the Society for Sociology at the University of Graz, Austria, on 2007, Retrieved on 2018.* THE GRAZ PAPER, 2018.
3. (a) W. Zuill, *Mob Programming: A Whole Team Approach.* AATC2017, 2017.

   (b) M. Hammarberg, *Mob programming – full team, full throttle.* 2013.

(c) Wikipedia, *Mobbing*. 2020. (https://en.wikipedia.org/wiki/Mobbing).

4. W. J. Dominey, *Mobbing in Colonially Nesting Fishes, Especially the Bluegill, Lepomis macrochirus.* Copeia, 1983. 1983(4), 1086–1088.

5. J. Kluger, *When Animals Attack — and Defend.* Time, 2007.

6. National Records of Scotland (NRS), *Index of Legal Terms - Mobbing and Rioting.* Court and Legal records, 2017.

7. N. Davenport, R. D. Schwartz, G. P. Elliott, *Mobbing: Emotional Abuse in the American Workplace*, Civil Society Publishing, 1999.

8. M. Mahmoudi, *BioImpacts,* 2019, 9, 129–130.

9. Seguin, E., *Academic mobbing, or how to become campus tormentors.* University Affairs, 2016.

10. K. Westhues, *The Envy of Excellence: Administrative Mobbing of High-Schieving Professors*, Tribunal for Academic Justice, 2005.

11. (a) K. Westhues, *Workplace Bullying in the Academic World?* Higher Education News, 2007.

    (b) M. Mahmoudi, *The need for a global committee on academic behaviour ethics.* Lancet (London, England), 2019. 394(10207), 1410.

12. R. McKay, D. H. Arnold, J. Fratzl, R. Thomas, *Employee Responsibilities and Rights Journal* 2008, 20, 77–100.

13. G. Namie, R. Namie, *Bully at Work: What You Can Do to Stop the Hurt and Reclaim Your Dignity on the Job*, Sourcebooks, 2009.

14. J. Towler, *Chaos and Academic Mobbing - The True Story of the Renison Affair.* John Towler, 2011, 78.

15. S. Khoo, *Malays Fam Physician* 2010, 5, 61–67.

16. https://www.insidehighered.com/

17. C. M. Crawford, *Confronting Academic Mobbing in Higher Education: Personal Accounts and Administrative Action*, IGI Global, 2019.

18. J. Harper, *Mobbed!: What to Do When They Really Are Out to Get You*, Backdoor Press, 2013.

19. K. Westhues, *Workplace Mobbing in Academe: Reports from Twenty Universities*, Edwin Mellen Press, 2004.

20. D. N. Walton, *Appeal to Popular Opinion*, Penn State Press, 1999.

21. J. E. Van Vleet, *Informal Logical Fallacies: A Brief Guide*, Hamilton Books, 2021.

22. Richard L. Epstein, *Critical Thinking*, Advanced Reasoning Forum, 4th edition, 2012.

23. H. Hansen, Fallacies, *Stanford Encyclopedia of Philosophy*, Stanford University, 2015.

24. S. M. Engel, *With Good Reason: An Introduction to Informal Fallacies* (2nd edition). New York: St. Martin's Press, 1982.

25. J. Earman, M. Janssen, J. D. Norton, eds, *The Attraction of Gravitation: New Studies in the History of General Relativity*, Vol. 5, Springer Science & Business Media, 1993.

26. H. Goenner, The reaction to relativity theory I: The anti-Einstein campaign in Germany in 1920, *Science in Context* 1993, 6, 107–133.

27. K. Hentschel, Albert Einstein: My Reply. On the Anti-Relativity Theoretical Co., Ltd. [August 27, 1920]. In: Hentschel K. (eds), *Physics and National Socialism, Science Networks. Historical Studies*, Vol. 18, Birkhäuser Basel, 1996.

28. Einstein, Albert Meine Antwort. Über die anti-relativitätstheoretische G.M.b.H., Berliner Tageblatt Volume 49, Number 402, Morning Edition A, p. 1 (27 August 1920), translated and published as Document #1, Albert Einstein: My Reply. On the Anti-Relativity Theoretical Co., Ltd. [August 27, 1920] in Klaus Hentschel (editor) and Ann M. Hentschel (editorial assistant and translator) *Physics and National Socialism: An Anthology of Primary Sources* (Birkhäuser, 1996) pp. 1–5.

29. S. Hawking, *A Brief History of Time*, New York: Bantam Books, 1998.

Chapter 6

What to Expect After Speaking Up?

Krzysztof Potempa

BRAINCURES Ltd, 2 Royal College Street, London, NW1 0NH, UK
potempak@gmail.com

This chapter outlines what to expect after speaking up against scientific misconduct that includes bullying, harassment, or discrimination. You will learn how to navigate the workplace grievance process, what the most common traits of "independent" investigations into allegations of workplace bullying or harassment are, and how to escalate your complaint internally and externally if you find the outcomes of internal investigation as biased and/or unfair.

6.1 Introduction

On January 15, 2020, the Wellcome Trust published a research culture survey of over 4000 researchers.[1] The survey revealed that:

- 43% of researchers experienced bullying, harassment, or discrimination in the workplace in the past 12 months,

A Brief Guide to Academic Bullying
Edited by Morteza Mahmoudi
Copyright © 2022 Jenny Stanford Publishing Pte. Ltd.
ISBN 978-981-4877-79-4 (Paperback), 978-1-003-16034-2 (eBook)
www.jennystanford.com

- 61% of researchers witnessed the above bad behaviors,
- 60% of the bullying was perpetrated by managers, and
- only 37% of respondents felt comfortable to report.

In response to the alarming degree of bullying, harassment, and discrimination of scientists by their senior mentors, certain members of the scientific community have (i) advanced seven principles to research culture change,[2] (ii) proposed that sexual harassment should be considered as research misconduct,[3] (iii) called for a ban on bullying in science stating that "institutions need to follow these policies to the letter, regardless of whether the alleged perpetrator is the director of the institute or a first-year PhD student, to protect all those involved—including the accused, who might be the victim of malicious allegations. Incomplete or unfair investigations can undermine the credibility of an organization, harm careers and signal to bullies that their behavior will be tolerated—in 2018 that is unacceptable,"[4] and (iv) proposed that institutions reputations should be tied to their anti-bullying records.[5]

6.2 Why Do Victims of Bullying Often Suffer in Silence?

In academia, thousands of bullies and harassers are institutional- ized (i.e., protected by the university). For example, Guardian's investigation into bullying, sexual harassment, and racial profiling at UK universities has revealed the following:

- There were 631 bullying complaints across 85 of 159 British universities associated with 300 people alleged to have bullied students and colleagues over a five-year period. Only 32 of the perpetrators were dismissed and 184 were disciplined.[6]
- There were at least 1953 reports of sexual misconduct committed by 1133 students and 264 staff at UK universities over a seven-year period. British universities then carried out 732 investigations resulting in at least 54 staff suspensions during an investigation and 20 were bans from teaching, which were both temporary measures.[7] Of note, an investigation by The Telegraph found that the number of sexual violence and

harassment cases against students in 2018–2019 had trebled to 1436, up from 476 in 2016–17, and that only 33 of the 124 universities used specialist investigators to interview students making claims.[8] Finally, the University of Cambridge received over 165 reports of rape and sexual assault over three years, and an ex-student Daniella Bradford is suing the university over its handling of her sexual harassment complaint.[9]

- There were 996 complaints relating to racial harassment against 461 students and 535 over a five-year period. Twenty Cambridge colleges provided inexact figures, while Oxford and Cambridge did not include staff complaints about students.[10]

The institutionalization of bullies and harassers, often referred to as the "pass the harasser" syndrome, is not just limited to the United Kingdom as:

- Michael Balter has catalogued hundreds of notable international academic bullies, harassers, and enablers since 2008.[11]

- The Academic Sexual Misconduct Database initiated by Julie Libarkin in 2016 contains over 1000 publicly documented resolved and ongoing cases of sexual misconduct perpetrated by U.S. faculty, administrators, and other staff. Users can search and browse the incidents by institution, person, outcome, and other data fields.[12]

- In 2015, the American Universities Climate Survey on Sexual Assault and Sexual Misconduct found that (i) 23.1% (every 5th) of female undergraduates had experienced some form of sexual misconduct, (ii) 10.8% (every 10th) suffered nonconsensual penetration—a figure that rose to 12.8% in the same survey last year, and (iii) low 5% to 28% reporting rates to campus officials and police.[13]

- In 2018, Revolt Sexual Assault, a graduate campaign group, and Student Room, an online student community survey, revealed that only 6% (every 16th person) reported sexual harassment, and the most common reason for silence was that the assaults were "not considered serious enough" by the victim.[13]

6.3 What Should Silence Breakers Speak Up About?

Based on challenge bullying and harassment guide of University College Union (UCU),[14] silence breakers speak up about negative managerial behaviors such as the following:

- Constant criticism of a staff member's professional competence
- Spreading stories and innuendo about members of staff
- Removing responsibilities from staff members
- Always giving the same staff member trivial tasks to do
- Shouting at staff in private and in front of colleagues or students
- Making threats
- Persistently picking on staff in front of others or in private
- Failing to include staff in meetings, briefings, and so on
- Obstructing professional development opportunities
- Blocking promotion
- Ignoring a staff member's views and opinions
- Belittling individual members of staff
- Constantly attacking a member of staff's personal standing
- Deliberately ignoring an individual's contribution
- Excluding individuals from work activities
- Adopting different rules for different people
- Excessive monitoring
- Excessive and unnecessary criticism
- Generating unrealistic expectations
- Regularly making the same person the butt of jokes
- Overloading and unrealistic work allocation
- Setting a person up to fail by giving impossible tasks or deadlines
- Failure to support staff having difficulty

6.4   What Holds Back Bystanders from Speaking Up?

If you ask Alexa, Siri, or Cortana **what happens when you speak up**, Google will give you five reasons you should speak up and advice on how to speak up when it matters. Interestingly, when you extend the question to "what happens when you don't speak up about bullying," Google top hits include why victims of bullying often suffer in silence and reasons why bystanders do not speak up. This difference in responses suggests that speaking up against bullying is a formidable task.

So, why do victims of bullying, harassment, or discrimination in academia opt to suffer in silence? One of the reasons is that researchers are quite concerned about reporting, as published accounts of survivors of bullying or harassment reveal that those who speak up are often left to rebuild their lives after they challenge bad behaviors by senior professors.[6] For example:

- Charlotte, a PhD student, recounted that following a miscarriage and then news that she is pregnant again six months later to her manager was met with the inappropriate statement: "Oh God, I can't believe it, this is going to be really damaging for your project. I actually thought that miscarriage you had was a good thing."

- A PhD student spoke of "abuse of power" by their adviser, which included "career sabotage, IP [intellectual property] theft and more general bullying such as belittling comments, often in front of or in response to senior academics."

- A junior staff member stated that their adviser "refused to give me any control over my own projects, and shouted things like 'I don't give a shit about your science' when I suggested improvements to experimental designs. I reported the abuse, but was told nothing would happen because he had just been given tenure and the university protects all their professors."

- A lecturer in social sciences at a different university described entering "a Kafkaesque nightmare" after making a formal bullying complaint against a colleague. It culminated in her being pushed to resign and sign a confidentiality agreement in exchange for a financial settlement.

- "They legally gagged me and threatened me."
- "Some students were driven to attempt suicide as a result, others broke down and simply vanished from science."
- "I lost my job, our entire family income and nearly my sanity. There are silenced victims like me all over the country trying to rebuild our shattered lives while the perpetrators carry on building their careers."

Similarly, survivors of sexual harassment have told BBC News[15] the following:

- Charlotte—not her real name—said she reported being sexually assaulted by another student while an undergraduate at the University of West London (UWL). "What happened after was worse than my assault," Charlotte said. She was "plunged into emotional chaos" and overdosed shortly afterward. She took three weeks sick leave to recover, but felt unsupported when she returned to university and her academic work suffered.
- Olivia, a student at a different university, was "bullied into keeping quiet." Her university threatened to sue her if she speaks out: "They told me to not tell my parents, to not tell my friends, to basically just be quiet about it... it made it feel like it was my fault."

Finally, those who have been gagged have told BBC News[16] the following:

- Anahid Kassabian, a former music professor at the University of Liverpool, said she felt like she was treated as a "burden" and "bullied out" of her 10-year job after being diagnosed with cancer.
- Another academic Amy, not her real name, says bullying sparked her depression; Amy's university had a fund to get rid of staff with "significant health problems."
- Emma Chapman, an award-winning astrophysicist, says she was sexually harassed by a man at University College London and received a £70,000 payout after a two-year legal challenge. Dr Chapman says the "trauma of the original incident is still there" with "nightmares of [her] house being set on fire." Shortly after her tribunal, she received several untraceable

voicemails of a person laughing down the phone in the middle of the night.

6.5 How to Report a Bullying and Harassment Incident?

The 2016 report on challenging bullying and harassment from the UCU contains the following model letter to report bullying and harassment to your institution.[14]

Model Letter to Report Bullying and Harassment

Your address

Their address

Date

Dear [manager as identified in institutional policy or more senior manager if a collective letter]

I am writing to register the following concerns which I believe are potential breaches of [the institution's] dignity at work policy [or other name for the bullying and harassment policy]:

List a summary of concerns either of the individual or a collective concern

Summarize some of the evidence [specific incidents or a survey]

I believe the concerns identified may be in breach of [the institution's] dignity at work policy. I believe the behavior complained of may also constitute a hazard which ought to be risk assessed under the [enter the relevant Work Regulation act, e.g., Title IX in the U.S. or Management of Health and Safety at Work Regulations 1999 in the U.K.] and its Code of Practice which requires an employer to identify a hazard which has the potential to cause harm or injury and assess the likelihood of such harm or injury arising from that hazard.

I believe that the actions of [individual manager or senior management if this is a wider problem] may constitute such a hazard and that the risks they may pose should be controlled.

I would appreciate confirmation that you will arrange a meeting in accordance with our dignity at work policy [or other name of the bullying and harassment policy] and that this meeting will consider my/our concerns and supporting evidence, and the health and safety aspects of our concerns. I would also appreciate if you could provide me with the monitoring information for the last five years [or for the period conducted] on bullying and harassment incidents within the institution broken down by department and by gender, ethnic origin, sexual orientation and disability of the complainant.

Yours sincerely

[insert your name]

6.6 What Cycle of Abuse Do Whistleblowers Often Experience After Reporting?

In a 2019, a survey of 399 whistleblowers conducted by All Party Parliamentary Group (APPG) revealed that 78% of respondents experienced retaliation and only 8% felt their company was generally supportive to their complaint.[17] The employee retaliation starts with relatively minor and informal retaliatory responses gradually that escalate into more serious and formal ones and often culminate in the departure of the whistleblower from the organization. The cycle of abuse ranges from isolation, scrutiny, counter accusations, disciplinary action, demotion/pay reduction, dismissal/forced resignation, nondisclosure agreements (NDAs), and ignored allegations or case dismissal following an independent investigation (see Ref. [17] for full details of what each stage involves). The following two selected case studies from the above report provide an example of what a whistleblower may encounter.

Case study 1: It seems like punishment

XX Ambushed my PDR with a senior manager unexpectedly being there and "sitting in" (2:1 dynamic, power imbalance). [Senior Manager] then harangued me and accused me of things I hadn't done, talked over me, badgered me, manipulated and misrepresented what I had said, breached my confidentiality, denigrated me, called me a negative and divisive influence in the workplace (because I had dared to raise concerns). [...] Lied to me, lied about me and lied about my team. Made it clear that as long as [senior manager] is in post she will block my promotion.

Suggested I will be moved and redeployed and my team broken up —
seems like "punishment." Over the following weeks when I said how
upset I was by this treatment I kept being given extra tasks to do but
no extra time to do it I ended up stressed, high anxiety, signed off sick.

Case study 2

The bank I blew the whistle to used 3 City law firms against me, 2 of
them 'Magic Circle'. The Global Head of Employment Law at one Magic
Circle firm claimed (in writing) that they *"had up to 37 people working
weekends on (my) case"*. I frequently had crates of documents sent to
my home after 10pm, on weekends and at the start of Public Holidays.
[lawyer] *"unintentionally omitted"* **over 95% of my evidence** from
the trial bundle they were ordered by the Court to produce, causing
a more than 6 month delay in proceedings. The [employers]' **lawyers
also lied to the Court** as to the relevance of documents (which were
unlawfully withheld) and **engaged in collusion in the production
of witness statements** which had bizarre, repeated errors across
multiple statements as to facts.

6.7 What Are the Most Common Traits of "Independent Investigations" into Scientific Misconduct?

A report on institutional responses to complaints in relation to sexual
harassment that was prepared for the 1752 groups in September
2018 states that most victims who seek justice are left disheartened
and shattered after speaking up against the institution[18]:

"I put my faith in the process, and I really regret having done that,
because they didn't get it right. They didn't have the requisite training;
they didn't have the requisite understanding. They were not capable of
making an assessment." Fiona, PhD student

The procedural failures that silence breakers need to brace for
include the following:

- Failure to include evidence/witnesses that a complainant
  puts forward

- Failure to adequately assess evidence with equal weight and on balance of probability
- Lack of expertise among investigators or decision-makers
- Processes that allow the staff member under investigation to sabotage the process or use it to continue their abuse. This could take the form of the staff member using delaying tactics to postpone hearings or meetings or using tribunal hearings to attack the complainant
- Getting the student or complainant themselves to contact other potential witnesses/complainants. This was used in one case as evidence of collusion by the complainants, which contributed toward the outcome of the investigation being overturned at the appeal stage
- Failure to share evidence equally with complainants/ witnesses
- Failure to inform witnesses/complainants that their evidence would be shared with the staff member under investigation
- Confusion as to whether interviewees were witnesses or complainants and lack of clarity around the rights of each
- Lack of communication from the institution to the complainant/witness
- Lack of support and advocacy from institution to the student
- Lack of legal support/advice for students/complainants

6.8 What Happens After an Independent "Scam" Investigation?

In one of the most epic research culture battles, the investigation led by partner Mary Jo White for which the University of Rochester paid $4.5 million to the law firm Debevoise & Plimpton in 2017 concluded "We ... do not believe that any potential claimant or plaintiff would be able to sustain a legal claim for sexual harassment in violation of [federal law]" into allegations of sexual misconduct by Florian Jaeger.[19]

The scam investigation by Mary Jo White resulted in a further nearly 2.5 year battle that commenced with the filing of 111-page discrimination lawsuit against the University of Rochester

(Dr Florian Jaeger, Catherine Nearpass, Dr Greg DeAngelis, Dr Robert Clark) as the whistleblowers Dr Richard Aslin, Dr Jessica Cantlon, Dr Celeste Kidd, Dr Steven Piantadosi, Dr Brad Mahon, Dr Ben Hayden, Dr Elissa Newport, and Dr Keteruh Bixby were not happy with the outcome. The battle opened with following letter that was sent to the University of Rochester's Board of Trustees:

September 1, 2017

Dear Members of the University of Rochester Board of Trustees:

It is with the deepest sadness that we have come to this point: the filing of a formal complaint with the Equal Employment Opportunity Commission ["EEOC"] against the University of Rochester [attached] for failing to act appropriately against a faculty member who has engaged in sexual harassment and has created a hostile environment for graduate students, and for retaliating against those of us who filed and pursued a complaint through university procedures. As the two senior faculty involved in bringing this case forward, we are also representing five of our junior colleagues and the many students who have been negatively affected by the events described in the EEOC complaint. Arriving at this point is especially tragic because it could easily have been prevented with appropriate action by the UR administration. Instead, the administration has inexplicably failed to defend its most vulnerable citizens—its students—and put future students at risk by failing to act appropriately on their behalf and it has retaliated against the faculty members whose only motive was to defend these students. Some of these actions by the University were illegal and others unethical.

To be clear, we take the present action because our experience with the current system for reporting harassment and retaliation revealed a university process that is biased and broken. Our concern is to identify and remedy the defects in how this matter has been handled by administrators and the repetitive failures of the University's offices of legal counsel, Title IX officer, and those responsible for investigating harassment and protecting victims. We want the university to support—not retaliate against—those who report sexual harassment and other acts that create a hostile environment for students and faculty.

For over one year since we first discovered the behavior of the faculty member in question, we have acted in good faith to follow the existing University procedures for filing a complaint, exhausted all appeals, interacted with every level of the administration, and hoped that in the end the University would do what the law requires it to do: ensure the safety of our students and the respectful treatment of our female colleagues. One of us met personally with President Seligman to explain why the UR legal office of counsel exercised bad judgment that put the President, the Provost, and the overall reputation of the University at risk. The response was silence. Then Provost Clark chose to double-down and praise the faculty member who was under investigation while chastising those of us who brought the case forward. Thus, after an incomplete investigation, internal examination, and attempts to force us to "move forward," the University chose to filter, distort, and cover up the facts, to deny the veracity of the complaints of 7 faculty members and 11 students, to disparage those of us who brought forward the complaint, and then to further retaliate against us when we refused to back down—all with the purpose of protecting a serial harasser, we assume because the University finds his conduct unobjectionable or does not have the will to take him on. Even a cursory review of our EEOC complaint will confirm that this characterization of the events is accurate.

There are a number of broader consequences of these failures. It is already widely known that the UR has condoned the harassing faculty member's behavior. That knowledge will become more widespread with the filing of our EEOC complaint and the resultant airing of these concerns in the press. The mishandling of this matter has resulted in the loss of some of Rochester's best faculty and will undoubtedly lead to more, as well as a loss of the ability to recruit the best faculty and students to replace them as this story spreads through the academy and the press. The University has lost key scientific grants due to these departures and will lose even more as additional faculty leave to escape the hostile work conditions and retaliation they have suffered, despite their efforts to protect UR, the department, and the student community they serve.

For those of you who do not know us, it is important to point out that we are not short-term faculty members who have an agenda to damage the University. On the contrary, we are two of the most loyal servants of the University of Rochester it has ever had. Together we have 57 years of service on the faculty.

- Both of us were department chairs (for a combined 15 years).
- One of us was Dean of the College and Vice Provost for Arts, Sciences and Engineering for 5 years.

- Both of us played central roles in establishing and building the Department of Brain and Cognitive Sciences (BCS)—the department that has been destroyed by this case.

- We both served many years on Faculty Council, Faculty Senate and Faculty Senate Executive Committee, the College Curriculum Committee, and numerous commissions and special committees.

- We both served on (and in some cases chaired) search committees for the president and other high-level administrative positions.

- We have been awarded honors from the University (Goergen Award, Garnish Award, Graduate Mentoring Award).

- Both of us are members of the National Academy of Sciences and the recipients of many other academic honors (with our departures, there are only 3 other NAS members on the UR faculty).

We are also experienced enough in administration to know what a University can (and should) do in cases such as these. That is why we are so profoundly distressed with the UR's failure to do what is right and with its effort to perpetuate a system that looks the other way when an egregious case is reported. Despite our best efforts, the present situation must be viewed as a colossal failure of UR leadership at all levels.

Here is what we are asking for:

- We want the University to take responsibility for its failure to protect victims and to reform its processes.

- We want public accountability that ensures that the system will work as it is supposed to and that those who come forward in the future to complain will be treated with respect, not retaliated against.

- We want the University to institute a comprehensive examination of its policies and procedures, using a set of external evaluators and benchmarks to ensure that in the future the University exercises best practices (and hopefully becomes a leader in setting the bar well above current standards). The outcome of this examination must be widely disseminated to ensure transparency and follow-through.

- Key among these changes is a revamping of the current system, which allows the counsel's office to represent simultaneously the alleged victim and the alleged perpetrator, while also protecting the University's interest in minimizing risk from whichever of these sides is judged to be more powerful. The current system clearly contains inbuilt conflicts of interest that beg for an adjudicator who is not beholden to the University administration and a victim's advocacy office whose job is to investigate, defend, and protect potential victims over alleged perpetrators.

- We want the University to formally apologize to the witnesses and victims and provide damage claims to those of us who have been retaliated against.

Sadly, the University has given us no recourse but to file the attached EEOC complaint. We understand that your first response might be anger at us for doing this. But we urge you to read the complaint carefully, to judge for yourself whether we have done the right thing and whether the University has or has not acted in ways that you are proud to defend. We believe that we have acted at every step on behalf of the University, its students, and the values that the law upholds and that bind us as a community. In light of our failure to achieve a proper outcome within the University, we view action with the EEOC as the best we can do to ensure that the University acts as it should, so that it will face the future with the highest values and with processes that adequately defend them.

We are ready to work with you to rectify the structural problems that exist at UR and to resolve this complaint quickly and decisively so that UR is protected to the greatest degree possible. We invite you to work with us to protect the university's legacy.

6.9 What Is the Future Outlook for Research Culture Change?

The University of Rochester Silence Breakers received a $9.4 million settlement in March 2020[19] after a further two-and-a-half-year battle. The settlement marked the end of a tumultuous episode that also drove University of Rochester's then president Joel Seligman to resign. It is the second highest settlement on the record since Dartmouth College paid $14.4 million to nine women who said they were raped, sexually assaulted, or harassed by three professors in its Department of Psychological and Brain Sciences.[20] The three professors Todd F. Heatherton, William M. Kelley, and Paul J. Whalen retired or resigned after Dartmouth moved to revoke their tenure (see #DartmouthDoBetter on Twitter). Further such chapter is captured within Michael Balter #STEMToo Rogue Blog.[11]

The scientific community must do better and together we must end bullying, harassment, retaliation, and victimization chapters as those suffered by the silence breakers described here. We can and must do kinder science.

References

1. Potempa K. (2020). The past, present and future of research culture. *LinkedIn*

2. Hunter J, McKernan R, Rankin S, Barroso I, Lechler R, Brady M, Rees G, Riley E, Stewart P, Teichmann S. (2020). Seven principles to accelerate research culture change in the UK. *Times Higher Education*

3. Marín-Spiotta E. (2018). Harassment should count as scientific misconduct. *Nature*, 557(7704):141

4. Ban bullying in science. (2018). *Nature*, 563(7733):600

5. Mahmoudi M, Moss SE. (2019). Tie institutions' reputations to their anti-bullying record. *Nature*, 572(7770):439

6. Devlin H, Marsh S. (2018). Hundreds of academics at top UK universities accused of bullying. *Guardian*

7. Batty D, Cherubini E. (2018). UK universities accused of failing to tackle sexual misconduct. *Guardian*

8. Turner, C. (2019). Sexual violence and harassment cases at universities treble in three years. *The Telegraph*

9. Speare-Cole, R. (2019). Former student suing Cambridge University over handling of sexual harassment complaint. *Evening Standard*

10. Batty, D. (2019). Which UK universities have received racism complaints? *Guardian*

11. Balter, M. A #STEMToo Rogue's Gallery of sexual harassers, predators, and bullies in the sciences. Retrieved from http://michael-balter.blogspot.com/2018/12/sexual-abusers-i-have-known.html

12. Libarkin, J. (2020). Academic Sexual Misconduct Database. Retrieved 08/15/2020 from https://academic-sexual-misconduct-database.org/

13. Proudman, C. (2020). Breaking the silence surrounding sexual harassment on campus. *The TLS*

14. UCU. (2016). Challenging bullying and harassment.

15. Croxford, R. (2019). Sexual assault claims 'gagged' by UK universities. *BBC News*

16. Croxford, R. (2019). UK universities face 'gagging order' criticism. *BBC News*

17. All Party Parliamentary Group (2019). Whistleblowing: The Personal Cost of Doing the Right Thing and the Cost to Society of Ignoring it

18. Bull, A. (2018). Silencing students: Institutional responses to staff sexual misconduct in UK higher education. *1752 group*

19. Wadman, M. (2020). University of Rochester and plaintiffs settle sexual harassment lawsuit for $9.4 million. *Science Magazine*

20. Hartocollis, A. (2019). Dartmouth reaches $14 million settlement in sexual abuse lawsuit. *The New York Times*

Chapter 7

Possible Solutions to Academic Bullying in Higher Education

Morteza Mahmoudi[a] and Sherry Moss[b]
[a]*Michigan State University, USA*
[b]*Wake Forest University, USA*
mahmou22@msu.edu

Unethical and inappropriate behaviors/actions, that is, academic bullying, in higher education is a rapidly growing and intersectional issue that affects students, postdocs, and researchers of all backgrounds and experiences. To truly create a safe environment in academia, all stakeholders including the scientific community, funding agencies, legislators, psychologists, institutions, and the public must address this problem in an integrated manner. This perspective focuses on possible integrated functioning solutions that all stakeholders can provide in a collaborative manner to reduce the incidence and consequences of academic bullying.

A Brief Guide to Academic Bullying
Edited by Morteza Mahmoudi
Copyright © 2022 Jenny Stanford Publishing Pte. Ltd.
ISBN 978-981-4877-79-4 (Paperback), 978-1-003-16034-2 (eBook)
www.jennystanford.com

7.1 Introduction

Workplace bullying has been considered in scientific research and discussions for approximately three decades.[1-7] Compared to various types of workplace bullying, academic bullying has received less attention for several reasons, including a lack of robust and comprehensive data on the incidence of academic bullying.[2,3,8-10] In recent years, however, various types of academic bullying in higher education as well as the economic, political, and social complexities of this unique bullying environment (often referred to as a "culture of cruelty"[11] and "mean and nasty"[12]) have been considered in more detail.[2,13-25] The unfortunate reality is that our current research environment favors the thriving of bullies.[23]

In contrast to the research on workplace bullying in business organizations, knowledge about academic bullying suffers from a paucity of robust data regarding the incidence of bullying for several reasons, including the lack of a safe and protective institutional reporting system for bullying incidents, fear of retaliation, and confusion over where to draw the line between academic bullying, academic freedom, and other appropriate interactional phenomena, including conflict, debate/critique, and performance appraisal. Despite the absence of robust data, some reports claim that academic bullying has higher rates than bullying in nonacademic settings.[3,23]

To understand bullying in the academic environment, we first need to define academic bullying. Although academic bullying in higher education constitutes a small portion of workplace bullying, it may have additional or different definitions that are unique to the academic culture and environment.[2,26] According to Einarsen and colleagues,[27] workplace bullying involves harassing, offending, or isolating someone or negatively affecting their work tasks in a regular manner (e.g., weekly) and over a period of time (e.g., at least six months). Academic bullying involves a wide spectrum of activities, some of which overlap with regular workplace bullying, including verbal abuse, public shaming, and isolation.[28] However, there are specific types of bullying that are unique to the academic environment, including inappropriate power of peers, violations of intellectual property, unfair crediting of authors, and even coercing lab workers to sign away rights to authorship and/or intellectual property.[20,23,29-31] Another feature of the academic bullying environment that differs from common workplace bullying is the large percentage of the international workforce in some countries. For example, the US has the largest number of international graduate students and postdocs.[32] According to the Project Atlas conducted by the International Institute of Education, more than 50% of US postdocs are international.[33] Cultural and language barriers, together with limited support from family and friends (which is the most frequently used way of responding to academic bullying[34-36]), may worsen the consequences of abusive behaviors compared to other types of workplace bullying.

Owing to rapidly growing scientific concerns about the incidence and severity of academic bullying in higher education, and its serious and growing effects on its targets and on scientific integrity, all stakeholders, including both the scientific community and the public, should act quickly and effectively in a collaborative manner to address this long overdue issue. We cannot place enough emphasis on the unique importance of integrated functioning of the various stakeholders in addressing academic bullying. Recent reports from the national academies of sciences, engineering, and medicine regarding the incidence of sexual harassment may help us to better understand the urgency of collaborative attention to address the issue of academic bullying in the most effective way. Although well-established policies and legal actions exist to address sexual harassment, a recent report from the national academies of sciences, engineering, and medicine revealed that there is no evidence in support of a significant reduction in sexual harassment incidents due to these policies.[37] The national academies of sciences, engineering, and medicine proposed that the culture and environment that currently supports sexual harassment should be changed to eventually enable us to significantly reduce incidences and consequences.[37] In my humble view, the lack of integrated functioning between relevant stakeholders is the underlying mechanism for the failure of the efforts to significantly reduce sexual harassment in academic science. In the absence of well-defined policies/protocols and regulations, one can imagine how severe the incidence and consequences of academic bullying would be. Below, we identify the main stakeholders and provide ideas about the possible integrated support they can offer to address this blight on the scientific community in a timely and effective manner.

7.2   Researchers, Writers, and Journalists

Researchers can conduct studies on incidences and types of bullying and publish their findings. Comprehensive examples of current reports from various universities and countries are summarized in a recent global review.[2] Writers and journalists can also report representative bullying cases; this increases awareness throughout both the scientific community and the public. Although the scientific community is well aware of bullying behaviors in higher education, public knowledge is mainly limited to school bullying; in other words, bullying in higher education is less publicized than school bullying. There are, however, several examples of these case report presentations by both scientific journals[16,18] and news-based magazines.[38-40] Increasing public awareness of academic bullying will create a better understanding of how it feels to its targets and thereby create a larger supporting force behind institutional reform aimed at creating safer environments for students and researchers. A couple of recent analogues of the important role of increased public awareness and its unique role in addressing (or facilitating the path to address) the issue are (i) Dr Clair Patterson's campaign that helped to address the vicious role of petrochemical industries in relation to toxic levels of lead[41] and (ii) the Green New Deal proposal and the youth activism of the climate school strike.[42] Another unique power of public awareness about academic bullying would be the ability to revisit the current "wrong" or inappropriate norms of academic culture and to create a clear and separated line between academic freedom,[43,44] other appropriate interactional phenomena (e.g., conflict, debate/critique, and performance appraisal), and academic bullying. Awareness of the serious and long-term psychological and physical side effects of academic bullying behaviors on targets (reviewed in Ref. 2) may have a preventive role among faculty who unintentionally engage in bullying behaviors due to the lack of clarity about the scope of behaviors considered to be academic bullying.

A meta-analysis on the global incidence of academic bullying and its consequences also suggests that the public should be considered a powerful, yet underutilized, player in academic bullying.[2] Public awareness may also be helpful in raising questions to legislators of various countries considering the limited available policy and regulatory solutions to the issue of academic bullying.[2]

7.3 Targets

Reporting the experience of bullying (which can be done at any time after targets feel secure enough to share these experiences with the public and the scientific community) is another important step toward better understanding the root causes and finding suitable solutions to academic bullying. It is noteworthy that in most cases, the outcomes of internal investigations by academic institutions (even when the bullying allegations were validated) are confidential for many reasons, including the protection of institutional reputation and the privacy of personnel records. When the outcomes are not publicly available,[14] there is no pressure for accountability on the members of the investigation committee to be completely unbiased and fair. The reporting of the experience of bullying increases the accountability of the investigation process and responsibility toward the outcomes at both personal and institutional levels. There are several good examples of self-reports of experienced bullying.[2,45,46]

Scientific publishers can play a key role in helping targets through recognition of specific journals that cover case reports of academic bullying in their specific field. The current science and case reports on academic bullying in various fields are mostly published in journals related to the social sciences. The impact and awareness of bullying in a wide range of scientific fields would be significantly improved if incidents of academic bullying in one field were published by related journals in their fields. For example, as leaders in the chemistry world, the American Chemical Society and the Royal Society of Chemistry could establish special journal issues that discuss bullying behaviors among scientists with chemistry backgrounds or validated incidents of bullying in chemistry (and related) departments. This approach would significantly improve awareness in specific scientific fields about the bullying problems in their own backyard, which would enable them to propose better solutions to address this issue that are more compatible with the culture and environment of their field.

7.4   Institutions

Although institutions are the first place to which targets of academic bullying can formally report, there is substantial evidence that a very low percentage of targets actually report their experiences to their institutions[34,35,47,48] (e.g., in some cases less than 2%[49]). There are several reasons for the lack of reporting, including fear of retaliation, mobbing, visa cancellation (for international targets), and the fact that institutions are viewed as ineffective in the fair/unbiased addressing of bullying incidents.[19,50-52] Institutions can create a trustworthy and fair/unbiased environment to enhance targets' motivation to report and can counteract academic bullying by establishing transparent, fair, reprisal-free, and publicly accessible reporting, including releasing the outcomes of their investigations.[19] One easy way to facilitate this process might be reporting a successful and fair investigation of a bullying report and the consequences to the target and the leader accused of inappropriate behavior (e.g., see the actions by the University of Adelaide against the outcomes of their investigation committee[53]). Of course, personnel laws in each country vary and in some cases may prevent this type of reporting, which is, in fact, part of the problem.

One of the major problems institutions may face during the course of an investigation is that academic bullies are clever. They know how to pressure students/postdocs over the phone or in private meetings to minimize the tracing of their actions.[20] When targets do not have documentation or witnesses to prove that they've been bullied, there is no tangible evidence that the bullying ever happened. In severe cases, unethical leaders force targets to sign away their rights to intellectual property and authorship.[20] Foreign scholars are more vulnerable to these actions due to their unstable visa status as well as their cultural and language barriers. In this complex situation, institutions need to create strategies to address these more sophisticated forms of false documentation. In addition to a well-designed training system for researchers, institutions can establish an investigation committee composed of people with multidisciplinary expertise, including psychologists and social scientists, to better examine documentation for signs of coercion or inaccuracy as academic bullies attempt to leave no trace.[20]

In the case that institutions validate bullying allegations against scientists, they should not easily grant them a second chance (even when they are star scientists[12] and bring significant funding to the institutions). In addition, institutions should ensure that they do not "pass the harasser" to another institution.[13]

Institutions also need to allocate specific funding sources to help the targets of academic bullying. One of the major issues that institutions currently face is the limited options they can offer to the targets of academic bullying. In addition, institutions should help targets to obtain the required resources to enable a "healing process," including psychological help, as there is evidence that unhealed targets may show abusive behaviors in their future careers,[54] mainly due to a strong positive correlation between enacted and experienced abusive behaviors.[55-60]

Anti-bullying policies are necessary regardless of the type and nature of the institution. However, due to the serious consequences of bullying behavior, some types of institutions have stronger policies than others. For example, it is evident that bullying behavior in hospital environments is directly related to medical errors.[61] To address this serious issue, the Joint Commission requires that all hospitals should have a code of conduct regarding disruptive behaviors.[62] The establishment of a similar code of conduct has recently been proposed for other institutions.[63] Although all institutions should have anti-bullying policies, institutions that are more prone to the emergence of bullying behaviors should be even more diligent about developing strict policies and regular monitoring systems. This is because laboratories in high-ranked institutions that may have a scarcity of lab positions,[64] low job autonomy, high workload,[65] and greater job insecurity[66] might be more prone to the emergence of bullying behavior than other labs in less prestigious institutions.[64] This is mainly because of the increase of (i) the "willingness to tolerate" abusive behavior and (ii) the "willingness to bully" by leaders in these institutions.[64]

Another critical and effective step that can be taken by institutions is to establish a robust system for assessing situational factors that may play a significant role in the occurrence of academic bullying, including but not limited to the emotional maturity/intelligence[67] and trait anxiety/anger[68,69] of lab leaders (i.e., how a leader is able to manage situations, control his/her emotions, and behave appropriately when dealing with lab members). The establishment of such assessments could help institutions identify leaders who might be at higher risk of exhibiting bullying behaviors, which creates a unique opportunity to supervise and train them to develop an acceptable degree of emotional intelligence, as well as appropriate ways to deal with frustration and anger, prior to the recruitment and hiring of (new) lab members. In addition, close and regular monitoring of high-risk leaders might minimize the occurrence of abusive behaviors.

Training and education of faculty members, students, postdocs, and staff regarding the concepts and differences between academic freedom and academic bullying is another critical role that institutions can play in reducing the incidence of academic bullying. Unfortunately, currently, the scientific community suffers from confusion about the concepts of academic freedom and academic bullying.[2] Academic freedom is the ability to express one's opinions and debate intellectual concepts without the fear of reprisal. Academic freedom provides a safe space to conduct research in any field and draw new conclusions. Although unethical leaders intentionally justify their inappropriate behaviors as academic freedom, there is a clear and intuitive line between academic bullying and academic freedom. Academic bullying occurs when leaders use verbal abuse, such as ridiculing students, public shaming, and isolation, silent treatment, and academic threatening, such as visa cancellation or providing a negative recommendation, in a regular manner and over a period of time. Debate and intellectual conflict can occur without devolving into ridicule, threats, and shaming.

7.5 Center of Excellence in Academic Bullying

The apparent prevalence of bullying in higher education necessitates a call to create a center of excellence to identify standard and universal definitions of academic freedom, appropriate academic behaviors (e.g., critiques and performance monitoring), and abusive behaviors. This is an essential step to create a robust and informative set of standards on academic bullying and remove any confusion on using academic freedom or other covers to justify bullying behavior. It would also help investigation committees to better understand the scope of academic bullying in order to better address the needs of targets and to discipline offenders. In the absence of well-defined and standard "terms" and "definitions" of abusive behaviors, identifying bullying behaviors is challenging, and the outcomes of meta-analyses of the current literature may be misleading. Such a center could provide standard protocols for the preparation of surveys consisting of well-crafted and psychometrically sound items[70] for targeted populations to maximize the robustness of outcomes. The use of such standard definitions and protocols would make future surveys more useful by creating a universal and dynamic library of research on academic bullying in higher education. Such information could help scientists in the field to better understand the root causes of academic bullying and enable researchers to propose possible solutions to minimize abusive behaviors.

7.6 Funding Agencies

Both researchers and institutions mainly operate through grants and awards provided by funding agencies. Therefore, funding agencies can assess the bullying records of researchers and enabling institutions before allocating grants to them. This strategy may also encourage institutions to improve their reporting system to be fairer and more unbiased toward the targets. A good example is the Wellcome Trust funding agency in the UK, which announced a new policy in 2018 which mandates that institutions report the bullying records of their grant applicants.[71] Institutions that fail (i) to consider bullying allegations in a timely manner and/or (ii) to report bullying behaviors to this funding agency will be banned from applying for grants.[71] Even funded projects can be revoked by the Wellcome Trust due to validated bullying behaviors (e.g., a US$4.5 million grant awarded to the Institute of Cancer Research in London was canceled[72]).

7.7 Global Committee

A global committee should be established that can access reports of academic bullying incidents in institutions and audit them.[73] Funding agencies may require certification from such a global entity to release grants to institutions. The global committee can be considered a center of excellence for the prevention of academic bullying. The standard protocols on how to report, investigate, and release the outcomes of bullying allegations by such an entity may provide a fertile opportunity to achieve robust and reliable academic bullying records and data. The emergence of such committees sends a signal to bullies that they are being held accountable and sends a signal to students and researchers that the environment is safe for them and that they do not need to tolerate abusive behaviors. A good example of such a global committee is COPE (Committee on Publication Ethics), which educates stakeholders on publishing ethics and provides protocols and strategies on how to report, investigate, and release the outcomes of allegations of scientific misconduct. More than 20 years of effort by COPE has made it a standard organization for publishing ethics, and almost all of the scientific publishers follow COPE's procedures for the ethics of publishing. Unfortunately, there are serious problems in fair and unbiased internal investigations of academic bullying incidents by institutions.[19] In the absence of a global committee to audit reports of academic bullying, institutions may not conduct unbiased investigations for several reasons, including attempts to protect their reputation, limited options to offer the targets, the bully's influence on the investigation, and the powerless nature of the targets.

7.8 Digital Identifier Agencies

Digital identifier agencies that recognize scientists and their works/research (e.g., ORCID) can provide a section regarding the bullying records of researchers. In the absence of publicly available bullying records, lab leaders with a proven history of bullying may move to a new institution without informing the new institution about their past conduct; this strategy may minimize the likelihood of "passing the harasser" from one institute to another.[13] The retraction of publicly available manuscripts due to scientific misconduct is a good example of how publicly available information enables new institutions to know about previous fraudulent scientific works by violators and minimizes the risk of "passing the fraud" from one institute to another.

7.9 Psychological Associations

Targets of academic bullying may face a wide range of long-term negative psychological implications, including depression and cognitive disruption.[47,74–77] Although psychological associations[15,78] and institutions/organizations[15,79] have made enormous efforts to address the psychological effects of workplace and school bullying/mobbing, the complexity of the environment in academic science and higher education (e.g., existing cultural and language barriers for international researchers/students/scholars) requires specific psychological knowledge and training. Therefore, psychological associations should comprehensively study the effects of academic bullying in higher education and train a new generation of experts with a deeper understanding of how to help the targets of such behavior.

Psychological knowledge in helping the targets of academic bullying has not yet been fully developed. The simplest analogy for this issue is the emergence of diseases related to e-cigarettes; a few months ago, the first death related to e-cigarettes was reported and confirmed in the US.[80] The issue is that, unlike traditional cigarettes, the type of lung diseases created by e-cigarettes are not known, and there are no established cures for them.[32] In the same way that researchers develop new protocols for addressing lung diseases caused by e-cigarettes, psychology researchers should develop new protocols and resources aimed a ameliorating the devastating effects on targets of academic bullying.

7.10 Legislators

The field of academic bullying urgently needs legislators to pass new laws regarding academic bullying. There is a significant effort in the US to pass bills on health in the workplace (e.g., efforts such as The Healthy Workplace Bill by Dr Yamada[81]). However, in addition to the difficulties involved in workplace bullying, the targets of academic bullying in higher education require additional considerations and regulations. For example, because a large portion of postdocs are international, they need to protect their visas from cancellation threats (which is the leverage bullies use to force them to use the code of silence against abusive behaviors) at least for the course of the investigation process. Through new laws, universities may implement the same zero-tolerance policy that exists in the event of sexual harassment once they know that their reputation is in danger and that they can be legally sued by the targets. Institutions may then provide training programs for both faculty members and students. In the presence of zero-tolerance policies, leaders dealing with unethical behavior are more alert to the consequences of inappropriate actions; therefore, the incidences of such behaviors should decline. To avoid confusion, we would like to emphasize again that these strategies would not be functional (as stated by the report of the National Academies of Sciences, Engineering, and Medicine for insufficient effects of regulations and policies on significant reduction of the incidences of sexual harassment[37]) unless all stakeholders work together in an integrative manner.

7.11 Policy Makers on Institutional Ranking and Individual Scientific Recognition

Decision-makers who design rankings can also collaborate in the battle against academic bullying by linking institution's reputation to their anti-bullying records.[21] For example, the industry-leading U.S. News & World Report, which ranks US universities and hospitals annually, can consider the anti-bullying records of institutions in their rankings. Although such rankings, for example, among hospitals, are intended exclusively to provide patients and their families with a data-driven decision support tool to help them decide where to seek care for specific illnesses and injuries, considering the anti-bullying record of hospitals is relevant because bullying causes adverse events, medical errors, and compromised patient safety.[62,82] Most of the top ranked hospitals are affiliated with prestigious universities, although they may have different research strategies and protocols than their affiliated universities, which benefits both parties (e.g., hospital researchers receive prestigious academic position, which helps them secure funding for the hospitals, and the universities send their medical students to the affiliated universities). Because their reputations are highly dependent on their revenue, we hypothesize that hospitals may have a greater tendency to cover up reports of abusive behaviors compared to universities. In addition to the hospital's reputation, a portion of hospital costs are covered by indirect funding costs that lab leaders bring to hospitals. These factors, among others, may force hospitals to have higher tolerance toward ignoring/covering up abusive behaviors. Declaring their anti-bullying record as a part of the ranking documentation may be an easy strategy to establish fairer and more unbiased investigations of bullying incidents in hospitals.

7.12 Conclusions

The central message of this chapter is that the establishment of collaborative strategies between all stakeholders in the academic bullying realm is critical to effectively addressing the growing issue of academic bullying at its root and ensuring that all bright minds can excel and progress. Although many of the proposed solutions have been covered by the current literature (reviewed in Ref. 2), the significant role of the interrelationships between stakeholders and the generative dynamics that their collaborative work can offer to diminish academic bullying has not been comprehensively addressed in the current literature (reviewed in Ref. 83). Although some of the proposed approaches in each category may seem like punishments to the bullies and their supporters, we would like to emphasize that the integrated functional outcomes of the collaboration between stakeholders would likely result in more prevention and less punishment. In other words, the integrated functioning of stakeholders may reverse the dynamic that effectively creates a factory of bullies and targets in the first place by reinventing our scientific culture and environment in a safer and more effective way. We believe that the proposed solutions and constructive teamwork between all stakeholders will enable the scientific community to minimize the incidence and consequences of academic bullying in their own backyards and create safer and healthier scientific environments.

References

1. Leymann, H. Mobbing and psychological terror at workplaces. *Violence and Victims*, 1990, 5(2), 119.

2. Keashly, L. In *Special Topics and Particular Occupations, Professions and Sectors*, D'Cruz, P., Noronha, E., Keashly, L., Tye-Williams, S., Eds., Springer Singapore: Singapore, 2019, DOI:10.1007/978-981-10-5154-8_13-1.

3. Keashly, L., Neuman, J. H. Faculty experiences with bullying in higher education: Causes, consequences, and management. *Administrative Theory & Praxis*, 2010, 32(1), 48.

4. Keashly, L., Harvey, S. Emotional abuse in the workplace. *American Psychological Association*, 2005, 201. Available at: https://psycnet.apa.org/record/2004-19514-009.

5. Keashly, L., Trott, V., MacLean, L. M. Abusive behavior in the workplace: A preliminary investigation. *Violence and Victims*, 1994, 9, 341.

6. Rayner, C., Keashly, L. Bullying at work: A perspective from Britain and North America, *American Psychological Association*, 2005, 271. Available at: https://psycnet.apa.org/record/2004-19514-011.

7. Harvey, S., Keashly, L. Predicting the risk for aggression in the workplace: Risk factors, self-esteem and time at work. *Social Behavior and Personality: An International Journal*, 2003, 31(8), 807.

8. Braxton, J. M., Bayer, A. E. Introduction: Faculty and student classroom improprieties. *New Directions for Teaching and Learning*, 2004, 2004(99), 3.

9. Norman, M., Ambrose, S. A., Huston, T. A. Assessing and addressing faculty morale: Cultivating consciousness, empathy, and empowerment. *The Review of Higher Education*, 2006, 29(3), 347.

10. Cameron, C. A., Meyers, L. E., Olswang, S. G. Academic bills of rights: Conflict in the classroom. *JC & UL*, 2004, 31, 243.

11. Zanganeh, S., Hutter, G., Spitler, R., Lenkov, O., Mahmoudi, M., Shaw, A., Pajarinen, J. S., Nejadnik, H., Goodman, S., Moseley, M., *et al.* Iron oxide nanoparticles inhibit tumour growth by inducing pro-inflammatory macrophage polarization in tumour tissues. *Nature Nanotechnology*, 2016, 11(11), 986.

12. https://www.nanomedzone.com/will-the-lessons-learned-from-cancer-nanomedicine-facilitate-the-clinical-translation-of-nanomedicine-beyond-cancer/

13. Mervis, J. Universities move to stop passing the harasser. *Science*, 2019, 366(6469), 1057.

14. Abbott, A. Germany's prestigious Max Planck Society conducts huge bullying survey. *Nature*, 2019, 571(7763), 14.

15. Duffy, M., Sperry, L. *Mobbing: Causes, Consequences, and Solutions*, Oxford University Press, 2011.

16. Else, H. Top UK genomics institute investigates bullying allegations. *Nature*, 2018, 10.1038/d41586-018-06131-8.

17. Hu, Y.-Y., Ellis, R. J., Hewitt, D. B., Yang, A. D., Cheung, E. O., Moskowitz, J. T., Potts III, J. R., Buyske, J., Hoyt, D. B., Nasca, T. R. Discrimination, abuse, harassment, and burnout in surgical residency training. *New England Journal of Medicine*, 2019. Available at: https://www.nejm.org/doi/full/10.1056/NEJMsa1903759.

18. Lewis, D. 'Paralysed by anxiety': Researchers speak about life in troubled ancient-DNA lab. *Nature*, 2019, 572, 571.

19. Mahmoudi, M. Improve reporting systems for academic bullying. *Nature*, 2018, 562(7728), 494.

20. Mahmoudi, M. Academic bullies leave no trace. *BioImpacts*, 2019, 9, 129.

21. Mahmoudi, M., Moss, S. E. Tie institutions' reputations to their anti-bullying record. *Nature*, 2019, 572(7770), 439.

22. Marin-Spiotta, E. Harassment should count as scientific misconduct. *Nature*, 2018, 557(7706), 141.

23. Moss, S. Research is set up for bullies to thrive. *Nature*, 2018, 560, 529.

24. Jackson, L. Reconsidering vulnerability in higher education. *Tertiary Education and Management*, 2018, 24(3), 232.

25. Pelletier, K. L., Kottke, J. L., Sirotnik, B. W. The toxic triangle in academia: A case analysis of the emergence and manifestation of toxicity in a public university. *Leadership*, 2018, 1742715018773828.

26. Braxton, J. M., Bray, N. J. Introduction: The importance of codes of conduct for academia. *New Directions for Higher Education*, 2012, 2012(160), 1.

27. Einarsen, S., Hoel, H., Cooper, C. *Bullying and Emotional Abuse in the Workplace: International Perspectives in Research and Practice*, CRC Press, 2003.

28. Tepper, B. J. Consequences of abusive supervision. *Academy of Management Journal*, 2000, 43(2), 178.

29. Tepper, B. J., Moss, S. E., Lockhart, D. E., Carr, J. C. Abusive supervision, upward maintenance communication, and subordinates' psychological distress. *Academy of Management Journal*, 2007, 50(5), 1169.

30. Twale, D. J. *Understanding and Preventing Faculty-on-Faculty Bullying: A Psycho-Social-Organizational Approach*, Routledge, 2017.

31. Jones, B., Hwang, E., Bustamante, R. M. African American female professors' strategies for successful attainment of tenure and promotion at predominately White institutions: It can happen. *Education, Citizenship and Social Justice*, 2015, 10(2), 133.

32. Giulimondi, F., Digiacomo, L., Pozzi, D., Palchetti, S., Vulpis, E., Capriotti, A. L., Chiozzi, R. Z., Laganà, A., Amenitsch, H., Masuelli, L., *et al.* Interplay of protein corona and immune cells controls blood residency of liposomes. *Nature Communications*, 2019, 10(1), 3686.

33. Rauch, J., Kolch, W., Mahmoudi, M. Cell type-specific activation of AKT and ERK signaling pathways by small negatively-charged magnetic nanoparticles. *Scientific Reports*, 2012, 2, 868.

34. DelliFraine, J. L., McClelland, L. E., Erwin, C. O., Wang, Z. Bullying in academia: Results of a survey of health administration faculty. *Journal of Health Administration Education*, 2014, 31(2), 147.

35. Senol, V., Avsar, E., Peksen Akca, R., Argun, M., Avsarogullari, L. Assessment of mobbing behaviors exposed by the academic personnel working in a university, in Turkey. *Journal of Psychiatry*, 2015, 18(1), 212.

36. Amur, S., Parekh, A., Mummaneni, P. Sex differences and genomics in autoimmune diseases. *Journal of Autoimmunity*, 2012, 38(2–3), J254.

37. Consensus Study Report. *Sexual Harassment of Women: Climate, Culture, and Consequences in Academic Sciences, Engineering, and Medicine*. The National Academies Press, 2018.

38. Mahmoudi, M., Lynch, I., Ejtehadi, M. R., Monopoli, M. P., Bombelli, F. B., Laurent, S. Protein–nanoparticle interactions: opportunities and challenges. *Chemical Reviews*, 2011, 111(9), 5610.

39. Hajipour, M. J., Laurent, S., Aghaie, A., Rezaee, F., Mahmoudi, M. Personalized protein coronas: a "key" factor at the nanobiointerface. *Biomaterials Science*, 2014, 2(9), 1210.

40. Foroozandeh, P., Aziz, A. A., Mahmoudi, M. Effect of cell age on uptake and toxicity of nanoparticles: The overlooked factor at the nanobio interface. *ACS Applied Materials & Interfaces*, 2019, 11(43), 39672.

41. https://en.wikipedia.org/wiki/Clair_Cameron_Patterson

42. Mahmoudi, M., Abdelmonem, A. M., Behzadi, S., Clement, J. H., Dutz, S., Ejtehadi, M. R., Hartmann, R., Kantner, K., Linne, U., Maffre, P. Temperature: The "ignored" factor at the nanobio interface. *ACS Nano*, 2013, 7(8), 6555.

43. Gabbert, M. A. The right to think otherwise, in *Academic Freedom in Conflict: The Struggle Over Free Speech Rights in the University* (Turk, J. L., Ed.), 2014. Available at: https://books.google.com/books?id=c-

NIAwAAQBAJ&pg=PA89&source=gbs_toc_r&cad=4#v=onepage&q&f= false.

44. Twale, D. J., De Luca, B. M. *Faculty Incivility: The Rise of the Academic Bully Culture and What to Do About It.* John Wiley & Sons, 2008.

45. Henning, M. A., Zhou, C., Adams, P., Moir, F., Hobson, J., Hallett, C., Webster, C. S. Workplace harassment among staff in higher education: A systematic review. *Asia Pacific Education Review*, 2017, 18(4), 521.

46. Hollis, L. P. *Bully in the Ivory Tower: How Aggression and Incivility Erode American Higher Education*, 2012. Available at: https://www.amazon. com/Bully-Ivory-Tower-Aggression-Incivility/dp/0988478226.

47. McKay, R., Arnold, D. H., Fratzl, J., Thomas, R. Workplace bullying in academia: A Canadian study. *Employee Responsibilities and Rights Journal*, 2008, 20(2), 77.

48. Minibas-Poussard, J., Seckin-Celik, T., and Bingol, H. B. Mobbing in higher education: Descriptive and inductive case narrative analyses of mobber behavior, mobbee responses, and witness support. *ERIC*, 2018. Available at: https://eric.ed.gov/?id=EJ1201843.

49. Zabrodska, K., Kveton, P. Prevalence and forms of workplace bullying among university employees. *Employee Responsibilities and Rights Journal*, 2013, 25(2), 89.

50. Kakumba, U., Wamala, R., Wanyama, S. B. Employment relations and bullying in academia: A case of academic staff at Makerere University. *Journal of Diversity Management (Online)* , 2014, 9(1), 63.

51. Lester, J. *Workplace bullying in higher education*, Routledge, 2013.

52. Cox, E., Goodman, J. Belittled: The state of play on bullying. *Australian Universities Review*, 2005, 48(1), 28.

53. Lewis, D. Head of prestigious ancient-DNA lab suspended amid bullying allegations. *Nature*, 2019, *572*(7770), 424.

54. Hershcovis, M. S., Reich, T. C. Integrating workplace aggression research: Relational, contextual, and method considerations. *Journal of Organizational Behavior*, 2013, 34(S1), S26.

55. Aquino, K., Tripp, T. M., Bies, R. J. Getting even or moving on? Power, procedural justice, and types of offense as predictors of revenge, forgiveness, reconciliation, and avoidance in organizations. *Journal of Applied Psychology*, 2006, 91(3), 653.

56. Detert, J. R., Treviño, L. K., Burris, E. R., Andiappan, M. Managerial modes of influence and counterproductivity in organizations: A longitudinal business-unit-level investigation. *Journal of Applied Psychology*, 2007, 92(4), 993.

57. Hauge, L. J., Skogstad, A., Einarsen, S. Role stressors and exposure to workplace bullying: Causes or consequences of what and why? *European Journal of Work and Organizational Psychology*, 2011, 20(5), 610.

58. Lian, H., Brown, D. J., Ferris, D. L., Liang, L. H., Keeping, L. M., Morrison, R. Abusive supervision and retaliation: A self-control framework. *Academy of Management Journal*, 2014, 57(1), 116.

59. Mayer, D. M., Thau, S., Workman, K. M., Van Dijke, M., De Cremer, D. Leader mistreatment, employee hostility, and deviant behaviors: Integrating self-uncertainty and thwarted needs perspectives on deviance. *Organizational Behavior and Human Decision Processes*, 2012, 117(1), 24.

60. Tepper, B. J., Henle, C. A., Lambert, L. S., Giacalone, R. A., Duffy, M. K. Abusive supervision and subordinates' organization deviance. *Journal of Applied Psychology*, 2008, 93(4), 721.

61. Wallace, C., Gipson, K., Wallace, C. Bullying in healthcare: a disruptive force linked to compromised patient safety. *Pennsylvania Patient Safety Advisory*, 2017, 14(2), 64.

62. Klein, S. L., Flanagan, K. L. Sex differences in immune responses. *Nature Reviews Immunology*, 2016, 16(10), 626.

63. Nik-Zainal, S., Barroso, I. Bullying investigations need a code of conduct. *Nature*, 2019, 565(7740), 429.

64. Mahmoudi, M., Moss, S. Scarcity of lab positions in high-ranked institutions creates a breeding ground for bullies. *BioImpacts*, 9(4), 251.

65. Baillien, E., Rodriguez-Muñoz, A., Van den Broeck, A., De Witte, H. Do demands and resources affect target's and perpetrators' reports of workplace bullying? A two-wave cross-lagged study. *Work & Stress*, 2011, 25(2), 128.

66. De Cuyper, N., Baillien, E., De Witte, H. Job insecurity, perceived employability and targets' and perpetrators' experiences of workplace bullying. *Work & Stress*, 2009, 23(3), 206.

67. Gibson, L. C. *Adult Children of Emotionally Immature Parents: How to Heal from Distant, Rejecting, or Self-Involved Parents*, New Harbinger Publications, 2015.

68. Hershcovis, M. S., Turner, N., Barling, J., Arnold, K. A., Dupré, K. E., Inness, M., LeBlanc, M. M., Sivanathan, N. Predicting workplace aggression: A meta-analysis. *Journal of Applied Psychology*, 2007, 92(1), 228.

69. Fox, S., Spector, P. E. A model of work frustration–aggression. *Journal of Organizational Behavior*, 1999, 20(6), 915.

70. Kahneman, D. *Thinking, Fast and Slow*, Macmillan, 2011.

71. Mahmoudi, M., Keashly, L. COVID-19 pandemic may fuel academic bullying. *BioImpacts*, 2020, 10(3), 139.

72. Else, H. Does science have a bullying problem? *Nature*, 2018. Available at: https://www.nature.com/articles/d41586-018-07532-5.

73. Mahmoudi, M. The need for a global committee on academic behaviour ethics. *The Lancet*, 2019, 394(10207), 1410.

74. Giorgi, G. Workplace bullying in academia creates a negative work environment. An Italian study. *Employee Responsibilities and Rights Journal*, 2012, 24(4), 261.

75. Singh, K. Measurement and assessment of bullying behaviours in departments and affiliated colleges of University of Delhi. *PEOPLE: International Journal of Social Sciences*, 2017, 3(2).

76. Yousef, H. R., El-Houfey, A. A., Elserogy, Y. M. Mobbing behaviors against demonstrators and assistant lecturers working at Assiut University. *Life Science Journal*, 2013, 3, 10.

77. Navayan, P. K., Chitale, C. A study of nature and prevalence of mobbing amongst teachers in higher education in Pune. *KHOJ: Journal of Indian Management Research and Practices*, 2016, 297.

78. Mahmoudi, M. A survivor's guide to academic bullying. *Nature Human Behaviour*, 2020, 4, 1091.

79. Mahmoudi, M., Ameli, S., Moss, S. The urgent need for modification of scientific ranking indexes to facilitate scientific progress and diminish academic bullying. *BioImpacts*, 2020, 10(1), 5.

80. Gewin, V. How to blow the whistle on an academic bully. *Nature*, 2021. Available at: https://www.nature.com/articles/d41586-021-01252-z.

81. Mahmoudi, M., Moss, S. The absence of legal remedies following academic bullying. *BioImpacts*, 2020, 10(2), 63.

82. Rosenstein, A. H., O'Daniel, M. A survey of the impact of disruptive behaviors and communication defects on patient safety. *The Joint Commission Journal on Quality and Patient Safety*, 2008, 34(8), 464.

83. Mahmoudi, M., Keashly, L. Filling the space: A framework for coordinated global actions to diminish academic bullying. *Angewandte Chemie International Edition*, 2021, 60(7), 3338.

Chapter 8

Epilogue

Morteza Mahmoudi

Michigan State University, USA

mahmou22@msu.edu

This short book is aimed to provide a brief, but essential, understanding of the academic bullying issue in the scientific community backyard, its root causes, and possible solutions that can be done by stakeholders to solve the issue, driven by (i) thousands of target stories which my colleagues and I reviewed in the past few years through our institutions' IRB approved global survey on academic bullying (https://papers.ssrn.com/sol3/papers.cfm?abstract_id=3850784) and (ii) the complaints submitted to the Parity Movement Organization (www.paritymovement.org).

In this epilogue, I provide some information about the type of helps that anyone at various positions can provide to help in diminishing this long overdue scientific issue.

As a student, postdoc, or early-career researcher/investigator, your very first step is to gather information about the ethics and interpersonal atmosphere in the new lab or work environment prior to signing your offer. It is much more likely that you will obtain

A Brief Guide to Academic Bullying

Edited by Morteza Mahmoudi

Copyright © 2022 Jenny Stanford Publishing Pte. Ltd.

ISBN 978-981-4877-79-4 (Paperback), 978-1-003-16034-2 (eBook)

www.jennystanford.com

accurate information from former lab members than current lab members, who may feel constrained from providing their honest input.

Based on the above information, if you determine that what you are experiencing is academic incivility, you can take the following steps to help yourself—and probably many others in the future:

- Take action against incivility earlier than later; if you tolerate incivility and adopt a code of silence, such behaviors may escalate over the time and give you more reasons to resort to silence, e.g., pending manuscripts and being closer to finishing your degree.

- Document every incident, as academic bullies work hard to leave no trace.[1]

- To ensure confidentiality, share your concerns with a university-based resource such as an ombudsperson, rather than a departmental resource. Ombudspeople are fairly independent (at least with regard to your department) and can offer you (i) advice on distinguishing between academic bullying and possibly misunderstood academic freedom and (ii) possible strategies for reporting and solving the issue.

- If you decide to report the case, it is crucial to create a "plan B," or exit strategy. This can significantly reduce the pressure you feel during the investigation process, which might be lengthened or compromised due for a variety of reasons.[2]

- Be alert against academic mobbing (ganging-up).

- Contact funding agencies and share detailed information about your case. Information on how to submit a bullying report may be available in the website of funding agencies. As an example, for US National Institute of Health (NIH), see the following link: https://grants.nih.gov/grants/policy/harassment/actions-oversight/allegation-process.htm

- Request a letter of summary from the investigation committee.[2] Such a letter will be helpful in protecting yourself for future jobs and prepare you to resume your complaint when you feel you have enough power and resources. The "me too" movement is a great example, as many former targets of sexual harassment finally had their voices heard.

If you witness incidents of incivility, report them to the available university resources (e.g., ombudsperson). Your reporting matters and can help reduce incivility!

If you are in a position of responsibility during an investigation of academic incivility allegations, you can do the following:

- Ask former lab members (rather than current members) to comment about the perpetrator. Although locating former members may be more difficult than simply asking current members, their feedback is likely to be more accurate, honest, and informative than that of current lab members, whose serious reservations might include fear of retaliation.
- Have a constant monitoring system to stop possible ganging-up and other types of retaliation against the target.
- Avoid unnecessary delays in the investigation process.
- Support targets during the course of investigation (e.g., separate targets from alleged perpetrators in the workspace to prevent possible retaliatory actions).
- Use the lessons learned from the "me too" movement and other institutions; the long-term costs of covering up for bullies may be much higher than facing the perpetrator.
- Remember that you are responsible for the larger goal of reducing academic bullying; if the perpetrator was found guilty, try to support the target and prevent the vicious cycle of innocent targets turning into future bullies.

If you are a part of the human resources team or decision-making committee responsible for following up validated incidents of academic incivility, you can have a strong influence on stopping the chain of academic incivility by:

- Keeping the shared information by targets fully confidential, until there is a clear plan/protocol on how to keep targets safe from possible mobbing and retaliation by perpetrators and their supporters.
- Informing the funding agency that supports the perpetrator by sharing the investigation outcomes. This is a straightforward way to avoid simply "passing the harasser"[3] to a different environment where they can focus on other targets.

- Make available to your community documented examples of the outcomes of your committee's investigation and actions, including discipline/punishment of the perpetrator and support to the target. This sends a clear message that your institution will not tolerate such behaviors and that targets need not tolerate incivility. Unfortunately, few institutions are setting good examples, instead sending mixed messages to both perpetrators and targets.

If you hold a position within a funding agency, require that universities report their anti-bullying records. Stop supporting perpetrators who have an established history of uncivil behavior.

If you work for an entity responsible for publishing university or hospital rankings, work to add anti-bullying records to ranking criteria.[4]

If you hold a position of responsibility in a national-level academy of sciences, verify that even "star" scientists in your membership maintain a record free of bullying. The latest efforts on ejecting a few members of National Academy of Sciences of the United States, with validated sexual harassment allegations,[5] is a suitable example.

Conclusion

Diminishing academic incivility in science requires attention and collaborative action by all members of the scientific workforce.[6] This commentary offers practical steps for various members of the scientific community intended to create a more safe and civil scientific environment for STEM and all other disciplines. Such an environment not only improves scientific progress and integrity, but also ensures that the same human rights in place outside the lab also apply inside it.The resulting safe environment can significantly improve scientific integrity. Last but not least, those of us who have experienced academic incivility know how excruciating it is to be a target, and how dreadful it is to fear retaliation that may put your life, family, and future career at risk. We cannot undo the bad behavior we experience, but surely, we can make the scientific environment safer for others. Always remind yourself that "as a human being, our average lifespan is only 3 billion heart beats; don't lose the beats in the hostile environment and protect yourself and your loved ones from regretting your inability to make changes to the galley proof of your life!"[7]

References

1. Mahmoudi, M. Academic bullies leave no trace. *BioImpacts: BI* 2019, *9* (3), 129.

2. Mahmoudi, M. A survivor's guide to academic bullying. *Nature Human Behaviour* 2020, *4* (11), 1091.

3. Mervis, J. American Association for the Advancement of Science, 2019.

4. Mahmoudi, M. and Moss, S. E. Tie institutions' reputations to their anti-bullying record. *Nature* 2019, *572* (7770), 439.

5. https://www.sciencemag.org/news/2021/04/national-academy-may-eject-two-famous-scientists-sexual-harassment.

6. Mahmoudi, M. and Keashly, L. Filling the space: A framework for coordinated global actions to diminish academic bullying. *Angewandte Chemie* 2021, *133* (7), 3378.

7. https://www.advancedsciencenews.com/you-are-not-alone/

Index

Printed in the United States
by Baker & Taylor Publisher Services